Reflexology and Associated Aspects of Health

A Practitioner's Guide

Reflexology and Associated Aspects of Health

A Practitioner's Guide

Adrian Seager

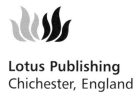

Lotus Publishing
Chichester, England

and

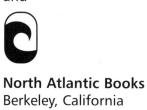

North Atlantic Books
Berkeley, California

First published in 2005 by
Lotus Publishing
9 Roman Way, Chichester, PO19 3QN and
North Atlantic Books
P O Box 12327
Berkeley, California 94712

Disclaimer

This publication is intended as an informational guide. The techniques described are a supplement to, and not a substitute for, professional medical advice or treatment. They should not be used to treat a serious ailment without prior consultation with a qualified health care practitioner. Whilst the information herein is supplied in good faith, no responsibility is taken by either the publisher or the author for any damage, injury or loss, however caused, which may arise from the use of the information provided.

Anatomical Drawings Amanda Williams
Photographs Chris Bromhead
Medical Photographs The Wellcome Photo Library
Text and Cover Design Chris Fulcher
Printed and Bound in the UK by Scotprint

Reflexology and Associated Aspects of Health is sponsored by the Society for the Study of Native Arts and Sciences, a nonprofit educational corporation whose goals are to develop an educational and crosscultural perspective linking various scientific, social, and artistic fields; to nurture a holistic view of arts, sciences, humanities, and healing; and to publish and distribute literature on the relationship of mind, body, and nature.

British Library Cataloguing in Publication Data
A CIP record for this book is available from the British Library
ISBN 0 9543188 8 9 (Lotus Publishing)
ISBN 1 55643 567 3 (North Atlantic Books)

Library of Congress Cataloging-in-Publication Data

Seager, Adrian M.
  Reflexology and associated aspects of health : a practitioner's guide / by
Adrian Martin Seager.
       p. ; cm.
  Includes index.
  Summary: "Written for practitioners as well as the general public, this book discusses a variety of
topics relevant to the practice of reflexology, such as coupling reflexology with complementary
practices, guidance on pre-treatment loosening techniques, dermatology, nutrition, meridians and
chakras, research, and treating stroke patients"--Provided by the publisher.
  ISBN 1-55643-567-3 (pbk.)
1. Reflexology (Therapy) 2. Alternative medicine.
  [DNLM: 1. Massage--methods. 2. Complementary Therapies--methods. 3.
Diet Therapy. 4. Skin Diseases--therapy. WB 537 S438r 2005] I. Title.
  RM723.R43S427 2005
  615.8'224--dc22
                              2005007281

Contents

Acknowledgements

A number of people suggested and encouraged me to write this book. Amongst the most enthusiastic has been Anthony Porter, to whom I owe my initial and advanced training in reflexology, and whom I thank for his permission to reproduce the summary of the various types of techniques of reflex contact for comparison in research (*see* Chapter 6).

Also, much has been learned from Dwight Byers, President of the International Institute of Reflexology and nephew of pioneer Eunice Ingham, and from Jan de Vries, a person of vast experience of the full spectrum of health and health maintenance, writer, broadcaster, lecturer and valued advisor. My gratitude to them both for their friendship, and for kindly writing the Foreword.

My grateful thanks to Gill Voisey for her patience and understanding in the production of the original draft and for being the 'foot-model' for the photographs.

To the late Harry Hawes, one time tutor at the Northern Institute of Massage; my admiration and thanks for some of the techniques illustrated in Chapter 2.

My thanks to the following for their invaluable help:

Jonathan Hutchings and Chris Jarmey of Lotus Publishing, for their patient help and guidance.
Keith Simmonds of Therapy World Ltd., for being instrumental in introducing me to the publishers.
Chris Bromhead for his photographic skill.
Amanda Williams for the illustrations.
Ros Ulderink of MR Publishing BV, The Netherlands, for permission to include '*A Basic Cellular Medicine Programme*' tabulation (*see* Chapter 4).

Loving gratitude to my wife, Norma, for quite simply, being there whenever a fresh shot of enthusiasm was needed to finish the work.

Finally, my sincere thanks to all my past patients – to whom this book is dedicated.

Foreword

About forty years ago, I met a gentleman in Ayrshire, Scotland, who had come back from the United States, and he gave me a glowing report on reflexology, and its benefits. I listened to him with great interest, as I had never heard of reflexology, to my shame. I decided then to look into the long history of reflexology, and discovered that it had been forgotten about for many years.

Only a few months ago, I attended a dinner. One of the guests was a very well-known professor of conventional medicine in London. During that dinner, he was asked what his thoughts were on reflexology, and I liked his answer. "There are many methods one can use to treat people, but it is wonderful if there are other ways that people can be treated without side-effects. I am certainly the last one who would say that there is nothing in reflexology. There is more to it that the eye can see." I was greatly encouraged by his words, as it was the sympathy of a man well known in the conventional fields of medicine who had opened his mind to what was there to help people.

I am greatly honoured to have been asked to do a foreword for this book, because when I started to study reflexology, and when deep in the background, I was disappointed to see how much scientific literature there was on this worthwhile field and today. This book by Adrian Seager, written with tremendous knowledge on the subject, which he now shares. What a marvellous book and so intelligently put together. I was very impressed but also very happy that at long last, in this field, we have a book so very much worthwhile.

Adrian has the knowledge but also the sympathy for patients who are eligible for this kind of treatment. It is therefore, not only for the person who wants to become a reflexologist, but also for the person at home that considers it. This book gives the help to understand this subject that is so often misunderstood, and with so many aspects to improve ones health.

I wish this book all the success it deserves and may the reading public find something within its pages to help them along and ease their suffering.

Professor Jan de Vries, N.D., M.R.N., D.Ac., M.B.Ac.A.

Adrian Seager's book demonstrates his sincere dedication towards the true meaning of reflexology. With this practitioner's guide, he brings better health to our fellow humans in a natural way.

This book is a must for all clinical reflexologists. It improves the application skills, which will enable the reflexologist to obtain faster and more efficient results. With this knowledge, one can add more insight to their skills to obtain better health on a higher plain of understanding reflexology in the field of science. The secret to becoming a successful reflexologist is through continued education and practise.

Adrian Seager is to be commended for his outstanding dedication to improving the knowledge and skills of the professional reflexologist and my sincere congratulations to Adrian for completing a book that every reflexology student should acquire for his / her library.

Dwight C. Byers, President and Founder
International Institute of Reflexology

Introduction

Numerous books about reflexology exist already. However a number of colleagues and friends over the years have suggested I should write a book and this is one reason for this one. The other reason is that, during my time as a practitioner and as a tutor, it was apparent that a 'partial vacuum' existed between qualifying and becoming established as an independent practitioner. It is a time when we are unsure whether we will succeed on our own. What if an unusual condition presents or an inquisitive patient asks a question I cannot answer? Later we wonder if there is more to our profession than we learned in our initial training. When we are established, curiosity takes over from self-doubt. But where can we find some answers to our curiosity?

This book is a contribution towards filling the vacuum by sharing experiences gained during a number of years in private practice – some of which were spent working alongside doctors in their health centre and some in training other people. Also, it is an opportunity to inform members of the general public of aspects of health maintenance – as distinct from the reaction to disease – by which time, sadly, it may be too late.

Continuous professional development programmes (CPDs) exist which are a great help. Indeed, attendance for a specified number of hours per year now forms one of the conditions of continued membership of the societies that, together, constitute the Reflexology Forum in the UK. In that respect, there is a gradual and determined move towards registration of a number of complementary therapies and it is encouraging to see the increasing momentum towards its achievement.

In my early days of practice there was a tendency to work on a patient by 'doing things' to the feet and hands. With time and experience, this mellowed both in intensity and in the duration of each treatment.

Initially, a treatment would take the best part of an hour; with practice and increased sensitivity of touch and its response, this time reduced to about thirty minutes without omitting any of the moves used previously.

With experience came the trap of presuming to know. It became a bad habit of jumping to conclusions, of listening only in part to what my patient was telling me. For example, if they were recalling difficulty in sleeping soundly, my mind would race ahead to the possibility of a heavy meal eaten too late at night, too much coffee, insufficient exercise, etc. This obscured efficient listening was precocious and impatient. It preceded the patient telling me of her concern about the wayward behaviour of her teenage son.

So we should not presume to know, let the body tell us via the feet and hands. Fine tune and do not bully the body by trying to rebalance everything at once. The body's energy is finite and, therefore, there is a limit to the pace and to the extent that it can progress towards homeostasis.

Experience taught me that least is best. Every body repairs or readjusts at its individual rate and we must recognise this and work in harmony with it. Consequently, in the latter years of practice, I might spend, perhaps, ten minutes only on treating the reflex areas that related to the patient's prime concern. Conversely, a few 'treatments' were 'therapeutic' listening for up to an hour – without even touching the feet or hands. The important thing was that these patients needed to tell someone who was not in any way connected with their life. Once they had got that off their chest we could begin the hands-on work at their next appointment, with the benefit of established empathy. Equally, once a patient's constitution had 'got the message' and there were signs that a readjustment was occurring, then the treatment could be more general and of longer duration.

It has been observed that a number of therapists (not necessarily reflexologists) set out to 'cure' instead of trusting the body's innate capability to respond, adjust and rebalance. Treat and stand back can be a very useful approach and is the philosophy of Bowen Therapy along with 'least is best'. The philosophy's merit is that it gives the body time; and time to register what has been done to it via the nerve pathways and interstitial muscular structure; time to readjust and to utilise residual energy – which might be significantly lower when they first attend for treatment. To allow time for the patient's body to adjust requires the trust and confidence in our ability that is built by experience.

The purpose of the book has been to provide a read as well as a reference into which the reader can dip from time-to-time. Equally, an effort has been made to simplify certain aspects that academics (particularly those in full-time research) seem to delight in complicating.

For many years there has been a plea for doctors and complementary practitioners to work together for the benefit of patients. At national level, the Prince of Wales' Foundation for Integrated Health is a focal point that is giving great impetus to progress towards this desirable state of affairs. Significant change often relies upon patient evolution and dogged determination and perseverance. So we should not expect rapid or dramatic changes; it takes time to convince sceptics and to mellow self-interest. However, it is helpful to understand the point from which our colleagues in mainstream medicine set out and this is the purpose of Chapter 1 (The Background to Some of Today's Health Care Practices).

Some of the excellent work of reflexologists and of those practicing similar therapies can be handicapped by insufficient or restricted circulation of oxygenated blood in and around the foot and ankle joint. To omit loosening the stiff, tense, foot and ankle is like working with the brake on. The reduced blood flow and trapped impurities would reduce the efficacy of the treatment. Encouraged by those with whom I have worked in this respect and to help overcome this restriction, a copiously illustrated number of loosening techniques is included. The intention is to provide a support and reference to practical training in these techniques. The content should **not** be regarded in any way as a DIY short-cut, because that would be very dangerous.

A reflexologist or physical therapist could be the first to encounter a skin condition and it is for that reason that an introduction to dermatology is included that outlines the more common conditions. They are comparable to those taught in a registered nurse's training. From a practitioner viewpoint, it is important to have sufficient knowledge to recognise a potentially serious blemish and to refer the patient to their doctor immediately. If in any doubt whatsoever, always refer.

Every day it seems that we read or hear about the latest research about some diet or particular food and its impact upon our health, either immediately or long term. A chapter on some of the aspects of the vast and complicated topic of nutrition, with sub-headings, acts as a quick reference. Those who wish to advise patients should gain a nationally recognised qualification. Otherwise, there is danger in a limited knowledge. It is an introduction only and is not intended, in any way whatsoever, as a source for prescription or to interfere with the advice from a medical physician, nutritionist or dietitian.

We all know that we rely on food as our source of energy, so it seems logical to follow a chapter on nutrition with one that addresses body energy in its various forms. It is intended to be sufficiently concise to be practical. The references at the end of the chapter provide a lead into more detailed treatment of the topic.

There is an increasing requirement to produce evidence-based data of the efficacy of a whole range of medical and other therapies. Chapter 6 recognises this trend and gives some guidelines for those interested in research projects.

An audit of work undertaken with stroke patients, together with the knowledge gained forms Chapter 7 and links with the previous chapter about research. Although the audit population was very small (too small for rigorous research purposes) there are some intriguing aspects of the outcome. Not least, that gradual recovery can continue long after suffering a severe and debilitating stroke. Its inclusion in this book is in the hope that others will be encouraged to do wider and disciplined research that would be significant and that would result in quicker and more thorough care and regard for stroke patients.

One of the most popular topics for discussion is how much pressure should be used by the practitioner? Should it be firm, light or somewhere in between? In Chapter 6 ('Research – Why and How?'), there is a summary of the various types and techniques of reflexology used by practitioners and recognised for their therapeutic value. This was compiled for the Reflexology Research Trust by my good friend Mr. Anthony Porter when we both served as trustees. Personally, a firm pressure was favoured but was not used exclusively. For example if a patient was very ill and of low energy, a gentle pressure was used and, in this case, for a short period of time only, i.e. 10 minutes, three times a week, I found to be more effective than treating for a longer period. As a generalisation, the pressure used was always adjusted to the patient's individual pain threshold and never exceeded.

This leads on to two other issues. One, the question of fees when asking, for best results, to see a patient three times a week. In my experience, this applied only when the patient's constitution was unlikely to cope with, say, half-hour treatments. In which case one fee only was charged, i.e. 3 times 10 minutes equals half an hour, so charge one fee only. It is for you to choose and to adjust to suit individual patient circumstances. It worked well in my practice. The second issue was that, quite often, qualified ex-students would doubt whether they could continue to practice because the therapy was damaging their thumbs. Without exception, this was because they had forgotten the importance, stressed during training, of using the wrists correctly – to increase leverage.

Another question asked of all practitioners, however long they have been in practice, is 'What conditions respond to reflexology treatment?' Because of its prime function of restoring balance to the ultimate, homeostasis, it is tempting to answer 'Anything!'

For the record, a summary compiled from over fifteen years of practice is included as an Appendix at the back of the book.

At the end of some of the chapters, you will find some links to further or more detailed work. Since this book sets out to bridge from newly qualified to the time it might otherwise take to gain experience, it seemed logical to avoid another partial vacuum of where to go from here. These links are only of those of whom I have had experience or who I know and respect. This can, therefore, be limited and an advanced apology is extended to any reputable individuals or organisations not given a mention.

It is hoped that these links, together with the 'Useful Addresses' at the back of the book will place it in a network of valuable reference and scope for advancement.

Throughout, the aim has been to write in a style that would interest not only reflexologists but would make an interesting read for a whole range of complementary therapists, both in the UK and overseas. Also it is intended for people who have experienced the benefits from other reputable complementary therapy practices and for those interested in the growing general acceptance of those therapies.

The overall purpose has been to focus on aspects, from my experience, that form a useful and relevant adjunct not only to reflexology but also to a wide range of therapies. Yet again, we must be conscious of balance – in this case to balance relevant knowledge that improves our overall effectiveness with avoiding becoming too general. I have seen a number of people dilute their effectiveness by letting their commendable curiosity and thirst for more knowledge lead them on a meandering, incoherent, path. Consequently, it becomes difficult for the general public to know what they offer or believe in. Given free choice it is up to each of us to decide whether to be specialists or generalists.

Chapter 1

The Background to Some of Today's Health Care Practices

Some of the ancient therapies such as acupuncture and a form of reflexology, for example, existed approximately 2300 BC. There is evidence of their existence this long ago in China, Egypt and Greece.

When we think of medicine and history, our thoughts turn to Hippocrates – regarded by many as the founder of present mainstream medical practice – circa 450 BC. Few seem to appreciate, however that he lived some 2000 years after some of these ancient therapies. Yet these and other complementary therapies are looked upon as latter day alternatives to the practice of allopathic medicine. In fact, they were the founders; it is mainstream medical practice that is the science-based alternative to ancient practices. In those days it was largely the use of herbs and natural remedies. In Europe, this was undertaken in a feudal system of 'medicine in monasteries' (approximately 400 AD). The wise man or priest was the teacher of his society, from which the name doctor has its roots: doctor means *teacher*.

One of the recognised giants of medicine was the French chemist and microbiologist, Louis Pasteur (1822–1895). Whilst not a physician, he was highly regarded in his lifetime and revered since his death as the scientist who pioneered bacteriology. He studied chemistry at the Ecole Normale Supérieure in Paris. Later, his curiosity lead him to question and to explore why wine and beer went 'bad' and milk went sour. To prevent this process, he developed a heat-treatment which we know as *pasteurisation*. His inquisitive quest and numerous investigations of fermentation lead to his conclusion of the presence of micro-organisms (microbes and germs).

These ideas were applied to medicine. Pasteur was convinced that the diseases of his time were caused by infectious bacteria which, prior to the invention of the microscope, were unseen. Nevertheless, he demonstrated that immunity could be bolstered by inoculation with a weak variety of the agent that caused the disease. Note the similarity with the philosophy of homoeopathy. Pasteur demonstrated the validity of his ideas by an anthrax trial, near Paris, in 1881. A control group of sheep, left untreated, died. Whilst those he had inoculated with his new anthrax vaccine survived.

His most spectacular success, however, was with rabies which remains a lethal disease. In July 1885, he treated successfully a boy named Joseph Meister who had been bitten by a rabid dog. The vaccine was adopted worldwide, he became a national hero, funds flooded in, and he was able to establish the famous Pasteur Institute in Paris. He was the founder of the science of bacteriology, rivaled perhaps, at least on the theory side, by the German Robert Koch (1843–1910).

After centuries of speculation it was accepted that contagious diseases were caused by living micro-organisms. Vaccination against the dangerous disorders, diphtheria and cholera, began. But it was not until the early 1940s that antibiotics became available in sufficiently large quantities (and the means of producing them in large batches were possible) that penicillin was hailed as something of a panacea in its time. Also, I remember there was M and B693 (sulphanilamide), but little else outside homoeopathic or herbal remedies and the caring family doctor was not so dismissive of any placebo effect.

Smallpox was another scourge across the world until the late 18th century and the pioneering work of the English doctor Edward Jenner. Two significant events far apart from each other, one in Constantinople and the other in Gloucestershire, UK, occurred at about the same time.

The first exciting response was not from a physician but from the wife of the British Consul in Constantinople, Lady Mary Wortley Montagu (1689–1762) who had been scarred by smallpox. She reported how Turkish women broke the skin and introduced minute amounts of infected matter. The purpose was to induce a mild dose of the disease that would give protection without the permanent pock-marking that was a feature of those who survived the disease. When an epidemic broke out in England in 1721, Lady Mary had her three-year-old daughter 'inoculated' and the practice spread.

Jenner used vaccination after noticing that, in Gloucestershire, it was common knowledge that dairymaids who contracted the benign cowpox disease from the cattle they tended were immune subsequently from smallpox. Consequently, he inoculated an eight-year-old, James Phipps, with matter taken from a cowpox pustule of a dairymaid, Sarah Nelmes. James developed a slight rash and fever but recovered in a few days. After what Jenner considered to be a safe period of time, he 'inoculated' James with a potentially lethal dose of the smallpox virus and it did not take – showing that he had been immunised successfully.

By 1799, Jenner reported that 5,000 people had been vaccinated against smallpox and Parliament rewarded him with a grant of £10,000. Vaccination against smallpox became compulsory in many European countries in the 19th century. In England, protesters argued that the state had no right to impose such medical intervention and won the argument. The disease was virtually eradicated throughout Western Europe by 1900 and the World Health Organisation (WHO) co-ordinated a programme of vaccination which lead to the elimination of smallpox by June 1979.

It is worth noting that there was a worrying outbreak in Britain in the early 1960s. I remember it because I was a suspected case until the local Medical Office of Health, called in by my doctor, confirmed that it was only a severe case of chickenpox. Also, the world's last reported case was in 1975 affecting a three-year-old Bangladeshi girl. Because bacteria and viruses seem to have a strong survival ability against some prescribed treatments, we would be wise not to drop our guard and to continue to improve and sustain everyday living conditions and good hygienic habits.

Before the work of these famous people, the first scientific advance of significance was the victory of *antisepsis* (the principle of destroying germs) and *asepsis* (the principle of the prevention of germs forming) that was, in many ways, the culmination of a long empirical development.

The first recorded practitioners of antiseptic chemistry were embalmers who preserved the dead bodies of animals and humans. Their methods may have been somewhat crude by present standards but they were successful to such an extent that mummies two or three thousand years old have been found with the soles of their feet still soft and elastic and with flexible joints! The preservatives used contained pitch, palm-oil, myrrh, cassia, cedar-oil and sometimes wax and honey. Alexander the Great, for example, was preserved in wax and honey[2]. The use of honey I find interesting because I know of cases of ulceration, for example, that have cleared with repeated application of honey under a sterile dressing.

Other instances of old antiseptic practice include the ancient custom of smoking fish and of salting pork (important in the pre-refrigeration days when embarking on long sea voyages).

In medical practice the growth of antiseptic methods was slow. Hippocrates recommended that wounds should be allowed to bleed freely and should be cleaned carefully. Similarly, Celsus made the same recommendation and suggested that a sponge moistened with wine and vinegar should be placed over wounds. Again, we see the present day use of cider vinegar either as a dressing which, when applied overnight to a sprain or similar injury, will reduce greatly the extent of local inflammation and swelling. Equally, it can be drunk to settle some kinds of digestive upset; farmers have long used cider vinegar to treat pigs that are ill.

Although Lord Lister was the first to recognise the surgical significance of the antiseptic theory and the first to appreciate the possibilities of carbolic acid, he did not establish the theory and neither did he discover the acid. To understand Lister's achievement, we must consider the development of antiseptic theory and the history of carbolic acid.

The theory of antisepsis and asepsis is based upon fermentation – the idea that all putrefaction is caused or processed by living germs.

In 1721, a Mr. Place observed and hypothesised that insects might be a contributing factor to the spread of the plague that was sweeping across Europe. If antiseptics could in some way exclude the insects from bodily contact, then this was promising material for medicine. He wrote: *"For the same virtues (antisepsis and asepsis) that preserve dead bodies from insects and putrefaction, I know no reason why they should not preserve living bodies from the same thing"*. Yet it was some time later that this idea bore fruit. What's new? We still have communication problems of this nature. Unfortunately, the spread and possible acceptance – or at least the proper consideration of new ideas – sometimes can be slowed by professional protection of the status quo. Little has changed.

The real seed of scientific antiseptic theory – based upon indisputable facts – was shown by Cagniard Latour's discovery that yeast contained living cells and that the fermentation of wine and beer was due to the chemistry of these cells. We have mentioned Pasteur's similar studies and theories. Whilst these developments were evolving, the theory of antiseptics was being established. Carbolic acid, the most significant of antiseptics, was being developed and its action upon suppuration was being studied.

Pitch, or tar, was one of the first known antiseptics and was used to preserve corpses and wine, and carbolic acid was a derivative of coal-tar. Even today we have coal-tar soap readily available although, it seems, not used quite as widely as in the 1960s.

In 1844, a Dr. Boyardee invented a powder containing coal-tar, sulphate of iron, etc. which he used to kill insects and to preserve wood. Maybe we should spray the roof timbers of our houses with coal-tar?

It was in August 1859 that Lemaire experimented with the use of coal-tar preparation in a case of gangrene. The results were significant and he continued experiments in other cases and finally, in 1863 – the date of the discovery of the first microbe of disease – he published his book on carbolic acid.

Lemaine was one of the great pioneers of antisepsis. He was a chemist who investigated the properties of carbolic acid (the constituent of coal-tar and discovered by Lange in 1834). As a thinker, he became aware of the antiseptic theory and saw the relationship between fermentation, suppuration, and disease. Yet he played a small part only in the practical exposition of the surgical possibilities of antisepsis.

Another pioneer of carbolic antisepsis was the Italian surgeon Bottini who, in 1866, published an article on the use of carbolic acid in surgery and taxidermy. Considering the number of cases Bottini treated, together with his evident grasp of antiseptic principles, he must surely share with Lister the honour of the practical application of the theory.

Lister started his immortal work in 1865. He was grateful to Pasteur whose research demonstrated the validity of the germ theory putrefaction. He acknowledged his indebtedness in 1874 – having proved antiseptics principles to the numerous cynics of his time. It is important to realise that in the 1800s was when it was common for 80% of wounds to become gangrenous; in 1868 the death-rate after amputation in hospitals was over 60%.

Some would diminish Lister's fame simply because others had carried out experiments successfully and previously when carbolic acid had been used upon wounds. But Lister's fame was not so much about the discovery of the antiseptic properties of carbolic acid as upon his conclusive demonstrations of its use in connection with disciplined antiseptic methods. Results were remarkable and account for his place in history.

At Glasgow Infirmary, Scotland, before the introduction of his methods, the death rate on its wards, post amputations, was 45.7%[2] compared with a fall to 15% during the first three years of his antiseptic treatment. From some of the horror stories that reached me when I was in practice, we would be wise to remind ourselves of the significance of disciplined antiseptic practice. This would include the utmost cleanliness of hospital wards at all times, particularly regarding keeping a watchful eye on visiting relatives and friends who nowadays drift in and out at any time in some of our hospitals. Nurses can be seen outside still wearing their uniform in which they return to the ward to continue their valuable work. It seems common sense to me to re-introduce forbidding that practice; one purpose of the uniform is as a barrier to unseen, avoidable, possible contamination.

Lister overcame opposition and sarcasm and won his argument. A scene familiar to many of today's would-be pioneers. He won, it has been suggested, because he combined science with art, had the courage of his convictions and the determination to succeed.

To me, the combination of science with art remains valid today. It is a vital aspect of health care and maintenance. If we can add some down-to-earth psychology, courtesy, empathy and humility (regarding the extent of our knowledge and experience) when "meeting and treating" – then we have a pretty good recipe for successful progress.

Smallpox was one of the great scourges of the 18th century and various ideas and methods were devised to try to contain it. We mentioned previously that inoculation was one method that was practiced in a primitive way. Basically, the technique was to break a pustule of an infected person, when it was 'ripe' and then to introduce the infected pus into a small incision – usually into the vein of an arm. The child, for it was usually a child, remained unaffected for about eight days before becoming poorly. Whereupon they were put to bed.

After pustules appeared – often as few as 20 – and cleared, the child recovered and enjoyed an immunity to the disease. Considerable debate ensued amongst the medics however. In those initial 8 days incubation a child would come into contact with many others who had no protection against smallpox and, as a consequence, would succumb and often die. Understandably, there was as much fear and opposition to inoculation as there was advocates for it. In addition, the poor living and poor sanitary conditions common at the time made infection of all types much more likely than they would be today.

So it was that some doctors – Dr. Wagstaff, M.D., F.R.S., of St. Bartholomew's, London, and Dr. Dolbonde of Boston, USA, for example, condemned the practice of inoculation as dangerous. Others, along with the general public, were in favour of the treatment.

After experiments on some charity children in 1722, the Princess of Wales had two of her own children inoculated against smallpox. Also, she persuaded the King to pardon some Newgate prisoners from the death sentence on condition that they would have to consent to be inoculated. Consequently, successful experiments were made on six condemned criminals.

Despite opposition, the practice made steady progress. In 1746 an inoculation hospital was established and eight years later the College of Physicians issued a statement in support.

There was no doubt that inoculation lessened the severity of smallpox but because no precautions against infection were taken, the disease outpaced efforts to contain it as each person inoculated served to disseminate the smallpox.

In a report of the diseases of London, 1796–1800, Dr. Willan quoted the case of a child that was inoculated in April and whose parents kept a shop that served about twenty local houses. The local inhabitants used the shop daily with the consequence that 17 of them caught smallpox within a fortnight and 8 of them died of the disease.

The average annual death-rate from smallpox for Europe was 210,000. During epidemics this rate was still higher. In Russia during one year alone, over two million died from the disease!

Dr. Lettson reported to a Parliamentary Committee that during 30 years preceding inoculation the death-rate from smallpox averaged 72 per thousand and during the 30 years following the introduction of inoculation it rose to 89 per thousand. The committee concluded that although inoculation preserved individual lives and more survived having contracted the disease subsequently, the general outcome was to spread and multiply the disease itself.

The missing link was a need for strict quarantine of those who had been inoculated during those critical eight days or so when the inoculated person was most at danger of infecting others. Such a precaution was advocated by Dr. Hayward in 1777. Unfortunately, unless and until the practice was widespread it was clear that individuals benefited at the expense of the majority. Consequently, its abolition would be for the greater good of the greater number. Indeed, in France and in Spain the practice of inoculation was suppressed. Whilst this was disappointing, the 'conquest' of smallpox was imminent.

Edward Jenner, the man whose work overcame Weil's disease, was born in 1749 at the vicarage in Berkeley, Gloucestershire, UK, and was inoculated against smallpox simply because it was in vogue at the time. He studied medicine under Dr. Ludlow, at Sodbury near Bristol, UK, and under John Hunter, in London, who is credited with stimulating Jenner's scientific zeal and research.

The idea that led to the successful combat of smallpox occurred by accident, although the first thoughts and curiosity had been kindled whilst he was at Sodbury. We owe the account to his biographer, John Baron.

Whilst at Sodbury, a young country woman consulted him and during the course of the ensuing conversation smallpox was mentioned. Whereupon she is quoted as saying: "*I cannot take that disease, for I have had the cowpox*". This comment stuck in Jenner's mind and when he went to John Hunter he discussed the issue with him. Subsequent enquiries amongst country doctors were inconclusive but Jenner remained curious and fascinated by the possibility of being able, perhaps, to vaccinate against smallpox by using the cowpox vaccine.

All cows at that time were milked by hand. Cowpox is a pustular disease of the udders of cows and caused sores to appear on the hands of dairy-maids when they came into contact with an infected cow.

Jenner experimented on his eldest son, then aged 18 months, with swinepox. He inoculated his son with swinepox initially and, at various intervals of time, with smallpox. The child, subsequently, appeared to be immune to the smallpox. But he could not be sure whether it was due to the swinepox or the follow-up smallpox inoculation.

In 1796, Jenner made his first significant experiment. He selected a healthy eight year old boy – James Phipps – whom he inoculated with cowpox taken from the sore on the hand of a dairy-maid. The boy developed a pustule on one arm and when, a few weeks later, he was inoculated with the smallpox virus he was immune to the disease.

Jenner wrote up his experience and in the very late 1790s sent the paper of the account of this case to the Royal Society, together with the conclusions drawn. It was returned to be published later under the long title of '*Inquiry into the Causes and Effects of Variolae Vaccinae, a disease discovered in some of the Western Counties of England, particularly Gloucestershire, and known by the name of cowpox*'. As far as is known, this was the first scientific attempt to make a connection between cowpox and smallpox.

Whilst Jenner may have been the first to take a scientific approach to the problem there is a suggestion that he was not alone in experimenting; some of which may not have been known widely. One such unofficial experiment was the best authenticated and most famous case of farmer Benjamin Jesty. There is conclusive evidence that, in the spring of 1774, farmer Jesty of Yetminster, Dorset, UK, worried for the safety of his family during an epidemic of smallpox, inoculated his wife and two sons with vaccine from his own cows.

Fifteen years later – in 1789 – the sons were inoculated for the smallpox by a surgeon from Cerne Abbas in Dorset, UK. This was together with others who had not received the cowpox inoculation previously. The arms of the two sons became inflamed but subsided quickly and they did not have a fever or suffer other adverse reaction. The others, however, had fever, eruptions and the reactions common to that time.

Farmer Benjamin's contribution is recorded as an inscription on a tombstone to be found in the churchyard of the village of Worth Matravers, near Swanage in Dorset, UK. Maybe a case of a layman who, by chance, anticipated the science. If so, how tragic that current medical hierarchy often appear to adopt an attitude of 'we know best' and can be very dismissive of the views of the layman or of the concerns of parents viz: MMR vaccination versus three separate jabs spaced at appropriate intervals of time that allows an infant's, as yet immature, immune system to cope with the challenge.

I recall, in the early publicity given to BSE how, when Professor Lacey suggested it could jump species – from animal to affect humans, his views were ridiculed. In fact, he seemed to be pilloried and, I believe, lost his job at the time. He certainly faded very quickly into the background.

He was, in expressing his opinion, threatening not one but two powerful interests; the meat industry and the suppliers of the organophosphates that were also coming under suspicion for a possible contribution towards the onset of the disease. This was a view echoed by farmer Purdey in Somerset, UK, who had observed his fellow farmers falling ill mysteriously after lamb-dipping and suggested that a possible link with the organophosphates used in dipping should be investigated. Time has proved the views of both of these gentlemen to have some validity.

To return to Edward Jenner (1749–1823) he championed vaccination against smallpox, from 1796 until his death 27 years later. But it was not without a fight or without his determination. Back in his day the world was afraid of new ideas and the practice of infecting a human with the disgusting disease of a cow was repulsive to many people; doctors wrote of grotesque facial features appearing on those who had had 'this dreadful' cowpox inoculation. A Mr. Ring claimed that his daughter, since inoculation, coughed like a cow. Others claimed to bellow like bulls. It appears there was quite an element of embellishment by those who opposed inoculation with cowpox.

It was against this atmosphere of opposition that progress towards the acceptance of vaccination was, inevitably, slow. In 1802 Jenner petitioned parliament to grant him remuneration for his discovery. The petition was referred to a committee which by a majority vote (three were against) granted him an award of £10,000, a large sum in those days. Even then the award was couched in words of caution and the battle continued between the pro-inoculationists and the anti-inoculationists. However, gradually all reasonable, rational, people were won over and rather like getting a boulder to the top of the hill, it gathers increasing momentum down the other side. So too did Edward Jenner's reputation and recognition gain momentum in line with the increasing widespread use of inoculation and its success in combating the serious illness of smallpox. He received the freedom of Dublin, Edinburgh and Glasgow and recognition from such diverse people as the Red Indians, Russians and Napoleon himself. Sadly, he died at the height of his fame, in 1823, of apoplexy (i.e. a stroke).

It is, perhaps, appropriate to put his achievement into the perspective of its time. The success of vaccination has made us forget its achievement. Today, smallpox has been reduced to an inconvenient illness rather than a threat. Although, of course, if it is caught by the unprotected it can still be lethal. Yet, in Jenner's time, it was a widespread disease right across the world that meant death, pain, deformity and blindness to millions of sufferers. It is against that grim background that Jenner's discovery and expansion of its benefit must be seen, despite prolonged opposition. We owe him a great deal of gratitude and his place in medical history is justified.

Anaesthetics

An antidote to pain has exercised our minds for generations. Equally, a definition of pain is the subject of debate that would keep undergraduates at their University Students' Union bar occupied for some time – until whatever they were drinking dulled their senses; a kind of layman's anaesthesia. We know it can be toothache, headache, earache, backache, haemorrhoids, muscle strain, bone fracture, etc. etc. but what exactly is pain? We could argue it's an electro-chemical signal along neuropathways from the site of some physical or physiological imbalance to a part of the brain that tells us it hurts. In this way nature ensures we stop, rest, etc. But prolonged acute pain can be very debilitating. In all these cases the need to suppress pain, or, even better, remove the root cause, is obvious.

So, historically, how did our predecessors combat pain? One drug used was Indian hemp or hashish that causes hallucinations of space and time – qualities that make it attractive to those who want to 'space-out' at the present time. In various nations, hashish was taken or prescribed before torture or death. It is claimed that a famous Arab chief drugged his followers with hashish so that they became incapable of fear or pain. The feats of these drugged followers – hashish eaters – gave origin to the word 'assassin'. It was sometimes inhaled and this may have been an early example of anaesthesia by inhalation.

Another drug used to deaden pain was mandragora of which Apoleius wrote, in 200 AD: 'If anyone is to have a member mutilated, burned, or sawed, let him drink half an ounce with wine and let him sleep till the member is cut away without any pain or sensation'. This suggests that mandragora, taken as suggested, caused the person to 'pass-out' with the unconsciousness being deep enough and long enough to overcome surgical pain.

Opium was another substance used to reduce pain by inhalation.

Mechanical methods were employed to induce insensitivity. In the 15th and 16th centuries it was discovered that humans and animals could be rendered unconscious by pressure on arteries carrying blood to the brain, i.e. the carotid artery. It was a method that was not used widely. Certainly it would have needed great care to avoid permanent brain damage from oxygen starvation to the brain.

The beginning of modern anaesthesia stemmed from the discovery of the beneficial properties of nitrous oxide (laughing gas) by Sir Humphry Davy. In the earlier days – late 19th century – a dentist, Dr. Riggs of Hartford, USA, pulled a tooth from a colleague (Dr. Wells) and wished to prove its efficacy, having heard of it via an exhibition in Hartford. Unfortunately, nitrous oxide has a transitory effect only and other doctors and dentists began a search to find a substance with a longer anaesthetic effect that would allow surgery requiring a significant time to be performed.

Two Boston doctors, Dr. Jackson and Dr. Morton claimed to have discovered the anaesthetic properties of ether and this lead to the controversy between the advocates of each technique. But, perhaps, the main issue was not so much about which doctor discovered the use of ether but who applied the discovery first. The literature gives that credit to Dr. Morton stating that he began his experiments in 1846. The first success was upon a spaniel dog, an interesting sequence of verification upon animals before applying the discovery to humans, much as we do with new pharmaceutical products today. Dr. Morton followed his experiment upon the dog by applying it to himself. He soaked his handkerchief in ether and succeeded in anaesthetising himself. Maybe the more pleasant effect of nitrous oxide – the laughing – would be a greater claim to any 'recreational' use. It remains for us to wonder and for them to have known.

I believe we owe a great debt of gratitude to the curiosity and courage of pioneering doctors like Dr. Morton. To give an idea of the risk he took, I can do no better than to quote from his report sent to the Academy of Arts and Sciences, Paris:

> "Taking the tube and flask, I shut myself up in my room, seated myself in the operating chair and commenced inhaling. I found the ether so strong that it partially suffocated me, but produced no deciding effect. I then saturated my handkerchief

and inhaled it from that. I looked at my watch and soon lost consciousness. As I recovered I felt a numbness in my limbs, with a sensation like nightmare and would have given the world for someone to come and arose me. I thought for a moment I would die in that state and the world would only pity or ridicule my folly. At length I felt a slight tingling of blood in the end of my third finger and made an effort to touch it with my thumb, but without success. At a second effort I touched it, but there seemed to be no sensation. I gradually raised my arm and pinched my thigh. But I could see that sensation was imperfect. I attempted to rise from my chair, but fell back. Gradually, I regained power over my limbs and full consciousness. I immediately looked at my watch and found that I had been insensible between seven and eight minutes."

I invite you, the reader, to put yourself in Dr. Morton's situation, alone, not knowing whether the experiment would work; if he overdid it, who would have found him and when? He experienced fear of whether he might die or ever recover his senses and the use of his limbs and even then not knowing if there would be a longer term adverse effect, mentally or physically – what courage!

Contrast this with today's insistence upon the need for 'scientific' evidence – double blind studies, etc. My fear is that the increase in litigation and, more particularly, the fear of it, will produce a whole generation of doctors who will only do that which is safe. So where will the future medical pioneers come from?

At the time of writing, there were two cases where the General Medical Council had called before it two doctors – ex NHS and now in private practice. One prescribed natural thyroxine, instead of the recommended synthetic product, and used tests for thyroid dysfunction that were in addition to the standard approved blood tests. The other doctor offered patients the choice of having their children vaccinated for measles, mumps and rubella (MMR) one at a time over an interval of time instead of a combined dose.

The MMR doctor was let off with a 'slapped-wrist'; the other was suspended for 'dangerous practice' – despite having helped thousands to an improved quality of life. Subsequently, he chose to retire in disgust. He suffered financial loss and his patients suffered the loss of the quality of life they had enjoyed under his care and diligence. How sad.

Each doctor, in my view, was doing no more than putting the patients' interest uppermost and, ironically, each had a record of thousands of successful outcomes. Yet they were victimised – reported by establishment 'colleagues'. Hardly an encouragement for future generations of doctors, who generally are trained to react to illness and disease rather than to protect and maintain good health. Overall, the greatest loss is not a threat to patient safety, but the loss of fairness and integrity.

To return to the tranquility of anaesthetics, Dr. Morton was the first to perform an operation under ether, as far as we know, without reference to practices of that era in the Eastern world – particularly the anaesthetising capability of acupuncture, for example. Apparently, Dr. Morton was given to elaborating his facts. So we must be careful of any sweeping claim. Yet he undertook anaesthetising a patient for surgical removal of a tumour at the Massachusetts General Hospital, USA, in the presence of sceptical peers. To do this dangerous experiment in such a public fashion meant Dr. Morton must have been a man of undying courage and self-belief. His whole career depended upon the success of the experiment, as did the life of the patient.

Summarising these developments, in 1844 it was Horace Wells of Hartford, Connecticut, USA, who established the anaesthetic properties of laughing gas (nitrous oxide) and two years later, Dr. Morton of Boston, probably encouraged or inspired by Dr. Jackson, also of Boston, established the anaesthetic properties of ether. I must, however, mention the humour of Oliver Wendell Holmes who suggested that statues of Drs. Morton and Jackson should be erected on the same plinth with the inscription "To E(i)ther".

Ether was first administered in England in a somewhat dismissive manner. Even today the established British medical hierarchy have great difficulty in acknowledging the research done by anyone outside the United Kingdom. It dismisses masses of anecdotal evidence with disdain and seems to regard only research undertaken by those attached to British Medical Schools as valid; irrespective of similar studies done in Russia, China or the USA.

The first operation in Britain under ether anaesthetic was witnessed at University College Hospital, London. Liston had consented to try the procedure, saying – it is claimed – *"Gentlemen, we are now going to try a Yankee dodge for making men insensible"*. The amputated leg fell to the floor in under one minute, prompting the further comment, *"This Yankee dodge, gentlemen, beats mesmerism hollow"*. Praise indeed.

Yet even these pioneers were overtaken by James Simpson, a baker's son and student at Edinburgh University Medical School. Witnessing surgery undertaken on a Highland woman (without anaesthetic) made a lasting impression upon Simpson. He was so appalled by the pain the woman suffered that he almost gave up his studies. Fortunately, he did not and vowed to search for some way of alleviating such excruciating pain. When ether was introduced he used it in obstetric practice but with limited success and continued his search for a substance that would have a more reliable anaesthetic effect.

He was a busy man with a huge practice, often not finishing seeing his patients until after midnight. Only then would he try various inhalants, assisted by his good colleagues Dr. George Keith and Dr. Matthew Duncan who also risked their lives.

They toiled unsuccessfully until one night in November 1847 when Dr. Simpson and his assistants tried chloroform. Briefly, the outcome was to experience euphoria – becoming bright eyed, very happy and very vociferous – followed by complete unconsciousness. Their initial experience was almost comical with all three men together causing chaos in their clinic as they were unable to control their actions as the effects of the chloroform wore off. Simpson had such a thriving practice that within weeks he had administered chloroform to over fifty patients and established to his and his assistants' satisfaction, its safety and reliability.

Even this significant discovery, however, was met with criticism, opposition and, one suspects, professional jealousy. It seems that human nature changes very little with time. So Simpson had to fight, as Jenner and Harvey fought, to convince mankind to believe the efficacy of his work and to accept the ensuing benefits.

One Irish lady confronted him claiming it was unnatural for doctors in Edinburgh to take away the pains of their patients! Dr. Simpson retorted that it was no more unnatural than for her not to have swum over to Scotland from Ireland, against wind and tide, but to have used a steamboat!

It was the theologians who were most opposed; to cause unconsciousness was seen as akin to witchcraft, one clergyman even claiming the chloroform was a decoy of Satan.

Dr. Simpson, for his part, answered all objections with patience, logic and wit. Today, we are so accustomed to the spotless modern operating theatres that we might fail to appreciate the significance of the work of Dr. Simpson and others of his era who lead the way.

We cannot consider the history of mainstream medicine without a mention of Pasteur and his contribution in the successful inoculation against rabies. At the outset of his work, no-one survived being bitten by a rabid dog. During a ten year period, 18,645 people were treated at the Institute Pasteur, with an average mortality rate of less than 5 per thousand (0.5%). Patients came from many parts of the world, including Brazil, Egypt, Greece, India and the USA.

To this day it is simpler to protect wounds from infection or to kill germs in accessible places than it is to rid the body of infectious diseases – tuberculosis, smallpox, malaria or typhoid, for example. Scrupulous hygiene at all times can minimise and confine an outbreak without necessarily overcoming it. These simple measures buy time in which we can introduce more significant procedures to overcome the disease – not least to boost the patient's immune system. Identifying the carrier has a vital part to play in the fight, for example, against malaria which is spread by the bite of mosquitos. If we can kill its larvae, we reduce the risk. If we can prevent TB patients coughing indiscriminately over others we decrease the chance of spreading the disease. These simple, self-help precautions have been known for years. But have we become complacent? If we had a serious outbreak of tuberculosis, where are the sanitariums into which we could isolate patients?

The advances in surgery have been profound. From being an adjunct to barber's shops to today's ability to transplant organs; sew back limbs by painstakingly joining blood vessels and nerve tissue; to joint-replacements.

At the beginning antisepsis was crude, such as Lister's cauterisation of wounds with raw carbolic. Anaesthesia was primitive and it was not unknown for patients to regain consciousness before the surgical procedures had been completed. Today, anaesthesia is a scientific discipline alongside other aspects of medicine. It needs to be to cope with the length of time the patient must be 'kept-under' and monitored throughout lengthy and intricate surgical procedures.

Ronald Campbell Macfie in his book, *'The Romance of Medicine'* (Cassell & Co. Ltd., 1907), records some amazing early procedures. Many fashionable people, for example, had their appendices removed at a time when surgeons had become quite blasé and opened the abdomen as a tailor might slit up a seam.

Dr. Harry Grey of Aberdeen, Scotland, opened the abdomen simply to squeeze the heart. He did this successfully on a woman, apparently dead or near death, having first slit her windpipe to alleviate suffocation. He inserted his hand, squeezed and massaged the heart and saved her life.

Whole stomachs were removed and the duodenum joined to the esophagus. Yet he writes that none of the patients without stomachs seemed to miss the organ and that some actually gained weight!

Significant heart surgery and repair was done in the late 19th century, notable by Pagen-Stecher, a well-known surgeon of that time.

The Duchess of Kent was amongst the first to have her hands X-rayed in 1896. X-rays enabled bullets to be located and removed surgically. Similarly, tumours could be located by the methods suggested by Galen and removed.

Latter day 19th century surgeons clipped off appendices, stitched up hearts, enlarged heads, curtailed intestines, transplanted skin and did some cosmetic surgery, such as straightened noses and smoothed wrinkles.

A history of medicine would be incomplete if William Harvey was not mentioned. He was born in 1578, gained an Arts degree at Cambridge, UK, in 1597 and studied medicine at Padua, Italy, where he qualified as Doctor of Medicine, in 1615.

When Harvey started his career, the teaching of Galileo maintained that blood and air passed from the lungs along the pulmonary vein into the left atrium. Harvey questioned this and eventually convinced his contemporaries that air was not passed along the vein but oxygenated blood (the exchange having occurred in the lungs) and that it was this oxygenated blood that passed into the lower left ventricle when the mitral valve opened as part of the heart's pumping cycle.

This proof arose because, quote: *"I profess both to learn and to teach anatomy not from books but from dissections; not from the positions of philosophers, but from the fabric of nature!"* So that when he divided the pulmonary vein, he found neither air nor vapour and so he asked: *"Why do we always find this vessel full of sluggish blood, never of air, whilst in the lungs we find abundance of air remaining?"* Furthermore, he demonstrated that even when the lungs were inflated artificially, no air passed along the pulmonary vein to the heart. His curiosity and enthusiasm to learn more about our cardiovascular system was born.

His surgical ability and investigations of the working of the heart destroyed the existing theory and beliefs. He then set about finding out how the heart did work. By using his astute and forcible logic, he eventually convinced the medical world that this vital set of muscles and blood vessels worked sequentially as we know it today – as an untiring, efficient, muscular pump.

The next puzzle was where did the continuous supply of blood come from and where did it go? On the one hand, it seemed veins would otherwise be emptied whilst, on the other, arteries would be filled to bursting. At the time, it was held that blood came from the juices of ingested food. Also, the belief was the blood moved only within the pulmonary system. Eventually, after much further and timeless work and using a great deal of determination needed to convince his critics, Harvey proved that blood circulated throughout the body, whilst simultaneously circulating around the pulmonary system. It is for this discovery that William Harvey rightly has a place in medical history.

Widening the View

Antibiotics are associated with current medical practice in the Western world. It comes as a surprise, therefore, to find that Egyptian physicians used them around 2500 BC by placing mouldy bread on wounds. The antibiotic (penicillin) was contained in the mould.

Similarly, we associate Sir William Harvey with the discovery that blood circulates throughout the whole body and was not confined to the pulmonary circuit. This was about the time of the Industrial Revolution in Britain; circa 1750/60. Yet the Chinese were familiar with the concept of complete circulation long before that era.

Even in the 5th century, India had civic hospitals where even the poorest were treated free of charge at the point of delivery.

In an attempt to put this summary of the history of medicine into a wider context, we will remind ourselves of the earlier physicians and of medical practice in the parts of the world beyond Western countries. This is a necessary part of understanding the fascinating, but very slow, progress towards an integrated medical approach to health or, in a wider context, to wellness.

The Hippocratic Oath

Hippocrates lived in the latter part of the 5th century and was a contemporary of Socrates. He was born in about 460 BC on the small Greek island of Kos. Strangely, there is no statue or bust of him that I recall seeing on the island, during a pleasant holiday in the 1980s, although there is a tree where he reputedly held counsel. Some years after his death, the library at Alexandria held a massive work called the *'Hippocratic Corpus'*. Alexandria had become a centre of medical learning and attracted physicians from Greece and Rome who continued their studies there. The massive work was very probably a compendium of numerous medical treatises and is regarded as an account of the work of Hippocrates, an icon – *'The Father of Medicine'* – leading to the ethical standard expressed in the Hippocratic Oath. Traditionally, the oath was incorporated into the graduation ceremonies of University Medical Colleges and read as follows:

> *"I swear by Apollo the physician, by Aesculapius, Hygeia and Panacea, and I take to witness all the gods, and all the goddesses, to keep according to my ability and my judgment the following Oath: To consider dear to me as my parents him who taught me this art; to live in common with him and if necessary to share my goods with him; to look upon his children as my own brothers, to teach them this art if they so desire without fee or written promise; to impart to my sons and the sons of the master who taught me and the disciples who have enrolled themselves and have agreed to the rules of the profession, but to these alone, the precepts and the instruction. I will prescribe regimen for the good of my patients according to my ability and my judgment and never do harm to anyone. To please no one will I prescribe a deadly drug, nor give advice which may cause his death. Nor will I give a woman a pessary to procure abortion. But I will preserve the purity of my life and my art. I will not cut for stone, even for patients in whom the disease is manifest; I will leave this operation to be performed by practitioners (specialists in this art). In every house where I come I will enter only for the good of my patients, keeping myself far from all intentional ill-doing and all seduction, and especially from the pleasures of love with women or with men, be they free or slaves. All that may come to my knowledge in the exercise of my profession or outside of my profession or in daily commerce with men, which ought not to be spread abroad, I will keep secret and will never reveal. If I keep this oath faithfully, may I enjoy my life and practice my art, respected by all men and in all times; but if I swerve from it or violate it, may the reverse by my lot."*

Aesculapius was an ancient Greek god of medicine. According to legend, he was the son of Apollo, and was trained by Chiron in the art of healing. He became so proficient that he not only cured the sick but restored the dead to life. Because Zeus feared Aesculapius could help people escape death altogether, he killed the healer with a bolt of lightening. Later, Aesculapius was raised to the stature of a god and was worshiped by the Romans who believed he could prevent pestilence. Serpents were regarded as sacred by Aesculapius and he is symbolised in modern medicine by a staff with a serpent entwined around it.

Hygeia was the Greek goddess of health. Her name is the derivation of hygiene; the principles and science of the preservation of health and the prevention of disease.

When we study the working of the Hippocratic Oath we can understand more clearly the behaviour of the medical profession as a whole and its reluctance to face some of the issues that have been forced into the open by the pressure of public opinion and action. The implications of the latter words are worrying and would be very applicable to anyone wishing to create or operate an exclusive and secret sect! You, the reader, must be the judge.

On a more cheerful and optimistic note, it is interesting to see how the Oath repeatedly refers to the practice of medicine as an 'art'. One wonders what the double-blind random control trial devotees make of that concept! In fairness, the reference to art may be a reflection of the time in which the Oath was framed.

The Oath certainly binds the profession into a closed family and it is easy to see how anyone who 'blows the whistle' is ostracized. Tragically, the whistle-blower may be doing no more than acting for the greater good of patients. To whom should such a person be loyal? To the 'club' or to the majority of patients? The answer should be obvious. In practice, it takes a brave, dedicated, practitioner to break ranks. Those who have done so seem, to me, to be those capable of thinking and acting solely in the interest of their patients; the entrepreneurs of the medical world. In placing them outside of the 'club', the profession does itself and us a disservice.

Perhaps Hippocrates' greatest contribution was that he separated medicine from the magic, religious influence and the superstitions mentioned previously in this chapter. He was a holistic practitioner. He proclaimed that disease was caused by the mental and physical state of the body and by its environmental conditions. Consequently, he took into account causes of illness both inside and outside the body. He regarded medicines as aiding the body's innate ability to heal itself. Sound familiar? It should, because it is the philosophy of present-day complementary therapies. Scientific medical practice seems to have forgotten its roots.

For a more comprehensive account of his work and that of Galen and Avicenna, I suggest you refer to Dr. Mosaraf Ali's book 'The Integrated Health Bible' (Vermilion, London, 2001).

It is sufficient for me here to mention Hippocrates' humoural medicine which consisted of four humours; blood, phlegm, yellow bile and black bile. He also recognised four types of human constitution; sanguine, phlegmatic, choreic and melancholic, depending upon which humour predominated. Notice the similarity with Ayurvedic medicine. It seems to me that all the various broad medical and therapeutic practices overlap whilst having a common aim; to alleviate or remove sickness and pain. They are like the tiles on a roof – they overlap at their boundaries when, collectively, protecting us from the elements (of illness). Singularly, they may be insufficient. Together, their effect can be profound.

Ayurveda Medicine

From Sanskrit, 'science of life', or 'knowledge of living', Ayurveda has its derivation of 'veda', meaning science, and 'ayur', meaning life. It is the traditional Indian medicine. The emphasis is upon health – maintenance – a more sensible and justifiable approach than reacting to illness. The latter is more painful and more expensive. Ayurveda concentrates upon the items, qualities and actions that can sustain us and warns us of those that can threaten to disrupt our health. Generally, it advises us about hygiene (cleanliness of self and surroundings) adequate exercise and a rewarding lifestyle leading to contentment. The emphasis is upon moderation and balanced diversity.

Gradually the widespread folklore in India was moulded into a more unified system at about the time of Hippocrates.

Dhanvantari was regarded as the icon of Ayurveda and whilst little is known of him, he is quoted often by physicians and writers. A compendium, similar to Hippocratic Corpus, laying out guidelines for the physicians' use of some 600 drugs in use at that time, was compiled by Charaka, whilst the surgeon Sushrat wrote a book based upon Dhanvantari's work and quoted inoculation via a scratch on the skin.

In 600 AD Vagbhata wrote a work of great significance, entitled *'The Heart of Medicine'* which was translated into a number of different languages. It contained a number of fascinating features, not least a seasonal regime in which the activities of people should vary in balance with the various seasons. I thought I had hit on something new because it is a personal view that we have much to learn and benefit from living with nature and the seasons of the year. He brought together a hitherto mish-mash of medical data and brought an order to it. Also, he identified over 100 reflex points on the body, similar to acupuncture points. Some of these points, or *marmas*, were lethal if punctured; others could paralyse and have become incorporated in some forms of unarmed combat. Others could be used therapeutically for disabilities and are still used at the present time by a minority of Indian practitioners.

Ayurveda encompasses a theory of Humours or *Doshas*; again notice a similarity with Hippocrates' philosophy. In Indian medicine there are three main Doshas. *Vata* (wind), *Pitta* (choler) and *Kapha* (phlegm), which are three constantly changing energy qualities that define all things on earth. They assist the practitioner to consider a patient's whole constitution, lifestyle, and environment as an integral part of diagnosis. Each is made up of a combination of two of the five great Elements of Ayurveda; Earth, Water, Fire, Air, and Ether.

Indians also established a link between these Doshas and the five senses. Kapha formed from Earth and Water, is linked with smell and taste; Pitta formed from Water and Fire, is linked with sight, and Vata formed from Air, and Ether, is linked with touch and hearing.

Kapha creates vital energy and affects reproduction, hydration and lubrication of the body joints, fat-regulation, the profile of body structure and protection against disease and ageing. According to Dr. Bagwan Dash (one-time official Ayurveda advisor to the government of India) Kapha is located in the lungs, and in the gastrointestinal system, at the level of the stomach and controls food absorption.

Some of the symptoms of Kapha dysfunction are:

• Loss of appetite
• Indigestion
• Excess mucus and its expectoration (bronchitis, asthma, tuberculosis)
• Excess fat
• Goitre
• Sensation of heaviness or numbness
• Heart and skin problems
• Obesity
• Anaemia
• Inflammation of veins

Pitta utilizes vital energy; assists oxidation, digestion, metabolic function, regulation of body temperature and vision. It is located in the small intestine, liver, spleen, pancreas and gallbladder. Some symptoms of Pitta dysfunction include:

- Excessive sweating
- Ulcers (of eyes, throat and mouth)
- Excessive hunger and thirst
- Fever
- Diarrhoea
- Skin disease
- Hepatic symptoms
- Bleeding

Vata controls the distribution of vital energy. It is involved with voluntary and involuntary muscle movement; breathing; the flow of vital fluids – blood, plasma, and the elimination of waste. Vata is located at the level of the large intestine. Symptoms of its dysfunction include:

- Digestive disturbances
- Gas and bloating
- Circulatory problems
- Headaches
- Agitation, anxiousness
- Insomnia
- Random pain that is difficult to locate

In the 14th century Sarngadhara wrote a book for the general public and, as a consequence, it enjoyed great popularity and remains available in some of the world's libraries. Many of his prescriptions were adopted by the pharmaceutical industry as recently as the 20th century. He wrote of numerous advances, including the medical use of opium and of the developments in inoculation. At the time of writing, there are moves in the UK to legalise the use of cannabis that is claimed to benefit those suffering neurological disturbances – particularly multiple sclerosis (MS). Whilst the debate regarding the safety, or otherwise, of combining inoculation against measles, mumps and rubella in a single dose continues, it just makes us realise the true pioneering significance and farsightedness of those tackling similar issues over 500 years ago!

Today, many colleges throughout India teach the Ayurvedic medical approach to health and its maintenance and it is formally recognised in that country and has the approval of its Government. To qualify to practice takes four years and includes anatomy, physiology, pharmacology, pathology, etc. All of which is comparable to Western 'conventional' medicine.

Traditional Chinese Medicine

Traditional Chinese Medicine (TCM), as the name implies, developed independently from Western medical practice. Successive Dynasties ordered the destruction of great swathes of recorded knowledge in their effort to expunge the past and to advance the dogma of their day. It is significant, therefore, that certain more permanent forms of writing survived and the need probably drove the method. One permanent method of writing was as inscriptions on bone or tortoiseshell. This was used in the Shang Dynasty from the 16th–11th centuries BC. They refer to diseases affecting the heart, head, intestines and stomach (which align with the four different fluids developed later).

The physicians, first mentioned in approximately 850 BC, had identified numerous seasonal diseases – including malaria in summer / autumn and coughing in winter. All were treated with herbs. They used four forms of diagnosis – inspection of the tongue; listening to a patient's voice tone and pattern, breathing, coughing; questioning the patient; feeling the pulses. Bamboo tubes were used as stethoscopes.

The use of needles to stimulate the body's energy lines (meridians) or to anaesthetise dates back to around 4000 BC. The analgesic effects of acupuncture gave Chinese physicians a great advantage over their Western contemporaries, particularly in surgical procedures although it is not clear whether instruments were sufficiently developed to take full advantage of these properties.

Probably the most famous surgeon of his time was Hua Tuo who lived in the 1st century AD (Han Dynasty). He was known as the 'miracle-working doctor' because of his mastery of many branches of medicine, including surgery, paediatrics, gynaecology and acupuncture. He performed numerous major surgical procedures using herbal anaesthesia. Also, he believed that the efficient circulation of blood was essential to sustain good health.

Another coincidence with the work and time of Hippocrates was the production of the Chinese medical classic *'Huangdi's Canon of Medicine'*, published between 475 and 220 BC; the time of the Warring States.

It was at about that time that the Chinese developed a humoral theory based upon four fluids in the human body; blood, phlegm, bile and black fluid.

The identification of Chi (Qi) – the body's energy source – and about which we hear so much today, occurred also at that period. They mapped its flow by careful observation of the reflex points used in acupuncture. According to Oriental philosophy, energy is the main element of humans and all living beings and is made up of two complementary poles, Yin and Yang – like opposite poles of a magnet. They were very aware of a person's temperature as well as their constitution and to this day still prescribe different herbs and strengths according to these two aspects. The work of the UK's Dr. Bach in the 1930s is similar to this approach and recognises the value of the delicate balance of physical and emotional wellbeing.

A classic on pulse diagnosis that exists still in China was Wang Shuhe's *'The Pulse Classic'* (210–285 AD, the Jin Dynasty). But the greater development of medical science in China occurred during the Ming Dynasty (1368–1644) and included the publication *'Prescriptions for Universal Relief'* by Teng Hong. It ran to 168 volumes and included numerous illustrations and over 60,000 prescriptions!

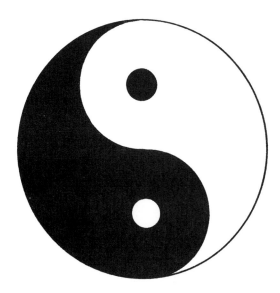

Figure1/1: The Yin-Yang symbol.

So What?

We can now appreciate the extraordinary similarity of some of the phases and developments of medicine quite independently and, in some instances, at about the same time in our history. I suggest the coincidences are sufficiently close as to suggest a degree of significance to present day challenges and that these coincidences would not have happened without some foundation for their collective validity. Yet Western medicine, certainly UK medical practice from the time of the 1939–45 War and onwards, has decried or been dismissive of much of this rich history.

Ever since the invention of the microscope, in about 1860, when we became excited about our ability to actually see the existence of microbes, we seem to have become preoccupied with a microscopic approach to health issues at the expense of considering the whole person; physical, emotional, mental, lifestyle. In short, to have the confidence and courage to use our eyes, ears, instinct and, above all, to *listen* to the patient whose opinions and concerns are too often dismissed as those of the unknowing simply because they have not had the opportunity of studying at a university medical school. There is a whole army of people well educated in other disciplines who are capable of thinking for themselves and who are gaining in confidence sufficiently to challenge some of the practices of mainstream medicine. A case of "It's my body, my life, we are talking about here, so please give me some logical reasons for your diagnosis, prognosis and prescription. Also, can you forewarn me of any adverse reactions I might experience as a by-product of taking the prescription?"

Many of us are quite capable of logical thought and our curiosity leads us to ask for explanations which practicing medics should have the confidence of answering, without fear of litigation.

If we know a little more about the origins of present day thinking and practice, we have a foundation upon which we can build understanding and mutual respect. I hope the other chapters, together, can form part of that building process.

References

1. Glanze, W.D. (ed.): 1998. *Mosby's Nursing and Allied Health Dictionary, 5th Edition*. London. (ISBN: 0 8151 4800 3).
2. Macfie, R. C.: 1907. *The Romance of Medicine*. Cassell & Co. Ltd., London.
3. Mosaraf, Dr. Ali.: 2001. *The Integrated Health Bible*. Vermilion, London. (ISBN: 0 09 185626 4).
4. Warrier, G., and Gunawant, D.: 1997. *The Complete Illustrated Guide to Ayurveda*. Element, UK. (ISBN: 1 8523 0952 0).

Chapter 2

Techniques for Loosening the Foot and Ankle

We have all encountered the 'concrete foot'. Usually, it is on the end of a patient that is tense by nature (often a perfectionist) or is suffering considerable stress in their personal and / or professional life. The degree to which reflexology can help is, to some extent restricted by this stiffness, certainly in the early stages of treatment. Some, if not all of this restriction can be removed initially with foot and ankle loosening. This increases bloodflow and the effectiveness of subsequent treatment, whether reflexology or massage.

This chapter gives an insight to some of these techniques. They span from those that are used by osteopaths to those that form part of the basic training of a qualified reflexologist.

The nature of this topic demands copious illustrations but you must appreciate the danger of using this material in a do-it-yourself fashion, because it is impossible in a publication to convey the vital feel, touch, force and co-ordination applicable to some of the moves. The moves shown as Part I would be reserved for qualified osteopaths, chiropractors and physiotherapists or for those who have attended seminars of content designed specifically to teach them and to oversee their application under observation and guidance. Attendees should be certified as competent to practice these techniques. Their use by unqualified / untrained people could cause injury. The reason for their inclusion is to give reflexologists an insight into what is possible. The photographs provide an aide-mémoire and reference. To those with whom I have worked over the years, they are a response to their request.

The reference numbers of the following sub-headed paragraphs refer to, and coincide with, those of the relevant photographs. A right-handed therapist is shown throughout.

Part I – Checking Existing Mobility

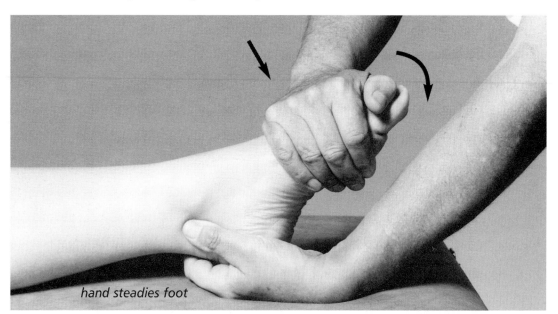

hand steadies foot

Figure 2/1:
Plantar Flexion.

The left hand supports and steadies the foot; the palm of the right hand is placed on the dorsal metatarsal area of the patient's foot. Applying gentle extension, the 'working' right hand bends the foot down; using sensitivity to feel and judge its full bend, whilst avoiding pain.

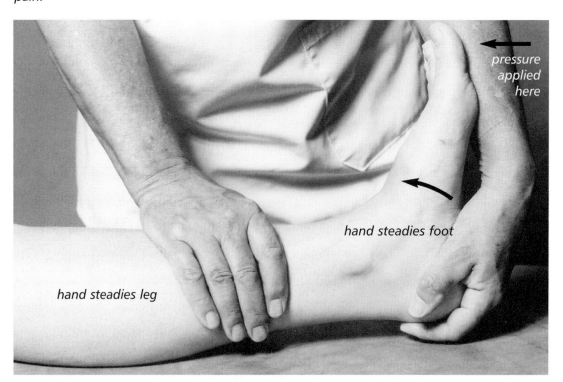

pressure applied here

hand steadies foot

hand steadies leg

Figure 2/2:
Dorsiflexion.

Left leg shown. Stand alongside leg and working from the lateral side, cup the heel in the left hand (as shown) so that the lower forearm rests against the metatarsal pad of the patient's foot. The right hand rests on the shin with sufficient pressure to steady the leg whilst applying pressure with the lower left arm up the leg towards the patient's head, as shown. Again, care is needed to feel and judge the 'stop' of the extent of full, painless movement.

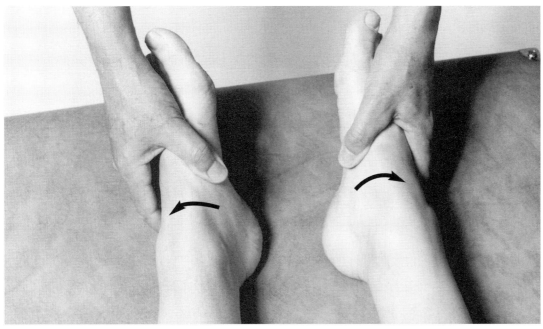

*Figure 2/3:
Abduction.*

Stand facing the patient and hold the patient's feet in each hand (as shown); rotate the feet outwards as far as they can be rotated without causing discomfort; make a mental note of the extent of maximum movement in abduction.

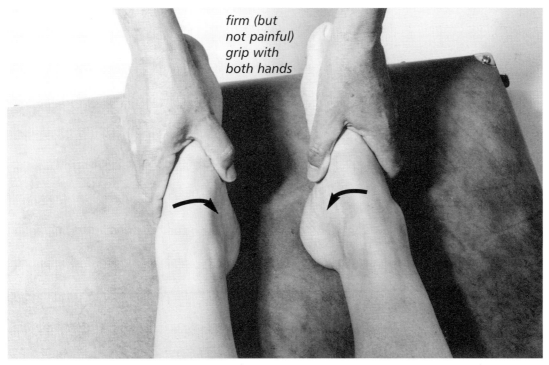

*firm (but
not painful)
grip with
both hands*

*Figure 2/4:
Adduction.*

As before, take the feet in each hand; this time, rotate them inwards, i.e. adduct the feet, to check their full extent of movement and make a mental note.

Continuing to Check Existing Mobility

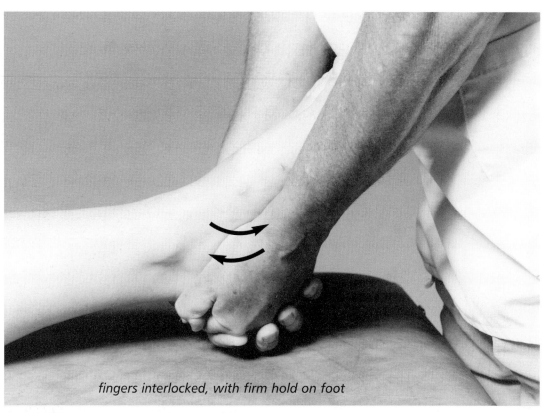

fingers interlocked, with firm hold on foot

*Figure 2/5: Rocking
Side-to-Side.*

Stand facing the patient. Take the heel (calcaneum bone) in cupped hands (as shown). Using a firm grip and fingers interlocked, turn the heel left-to-right and back again; in a horizontal plane. Repeat movement three or four times or until some extra movement is felt. But remember that the purpose of the move, primarily, is to judge existing mobility without pain.

Existing Mobility Concluded

Part II – Loosening the Foot and Ankle

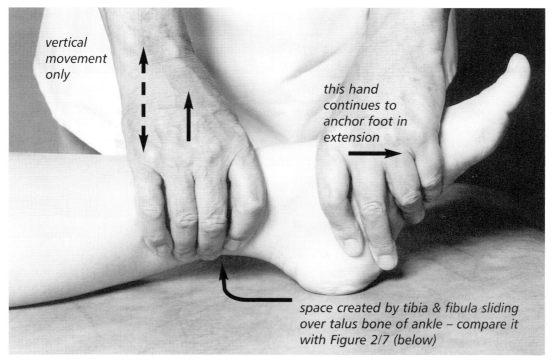

vertical movement only

this hand continues to anchor foot in extension

space created by tibia & fibula sliding over talus bone of ankle – compare it with Figure 2/7 (below)

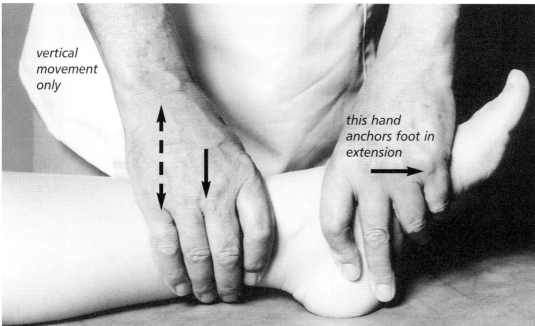

vertical movement only

this hand anchors foot in extension

Figures 2/6 & 2/7: Talus Loosening.

This move is to enable the joint formed between the tibia and fibula (that straddle the talus bone) to slide freely. The left hand grips the foot sufficiently to maintain the whole joint in extension whilst the primary movements are made. The 'working' right hand folds over the lower leg, above and adjacent to, the malleoli (as shown) and grips it sufficiently to lift it vertically whilst the left hand anchors the foot. Repeat the vertical up-and-down movement until increased, sliding movement is felt; probably after a minimum of five / six movements but no more than seven or eight. Take great care to ensure the grip used by the right hand does not pinch or cause the patient unnecessary discomfort and that the movement of the hand remains vertical throughout.

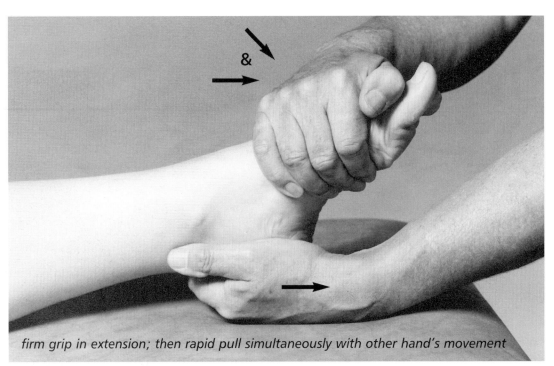

firm grip in extension; then rapid pull simultaneously with other hand's movement

Figure 2/8: Talus Separation.

Grasp the heel with the left hand, place the right hand on the dorsal surface of the foot. Apply extension with both hands (slight pull) before applying a rapid pull and abrupt downward pull (right hand) simultaneously; as if pulling the foot off the leg. **Not to be attempted on patients with a hip problem or replacement hip joint**. Care and feel needed at all times.

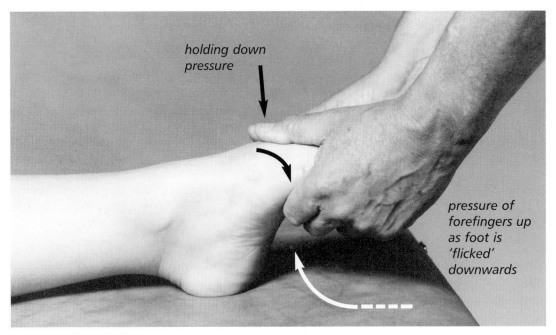

holding down pressure

pressure of forefingers up as foot is 'flicked' downwards

Figure 2/9: Loosening Cuneiform Bones.

Place the inner border of the forefingers under the area of the cuboid bones. Apply traction and a rapid movement of fingers upwards as thumbs press down simultaneously; to break adhesions. Repeat a few times, working across foot and a little towards the toes. Once again, practise is needed to get this co-ordinated 'flick' correct and to avoid injury.

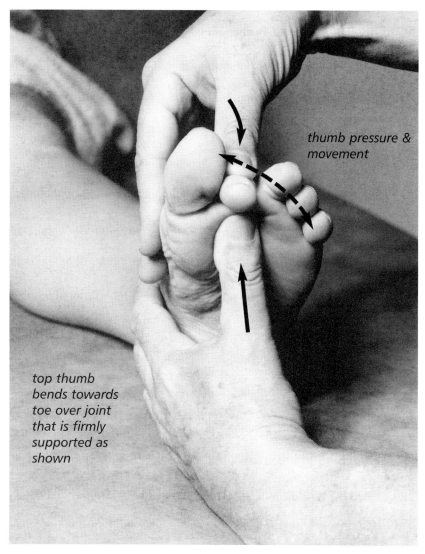

thumb pressure & movement

top thumb bends towards toe over joint that is firmly supported as shown

Figure 2/10: Loosening Metatarsophalangeal Joint of Small Toes.

Note: This move must never be done on the big toe (hallux) which has a saddle joint. *On small toes only, it is excellent for loosening the joints. Use whichever thumb above the toe that feels comfortable. Here, the thumb of the right hand is above; the thumb of the left hand supports the respective metatarsal joint and opposes the downward thrust of the right thumb. The 'slack' movement is taken up before applying rapid downward pressure at the same time as the supporting thumb gives a small upward, opposing, thrust. Repeat across the foot on each of the four joints, in turn. Often a slight popping sound accompanies the move, as the joint's partial vacuum is released. But this does not have to happen for the toes to be loosened.*

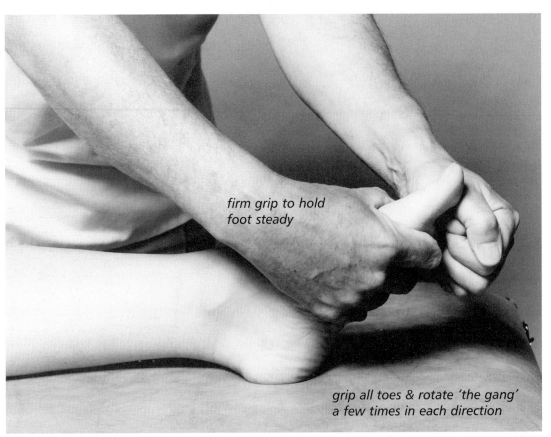

firm grip to hold
foot steady

grip all toes & rotate 'the gang'
a few times in each direction

Figure 2/11:
Collective Loosening
of Small Toes.

Stand alongside the leg and grip all the small toes (not big-toe) in a fist of the left hand (as shown). Rotate the collective 'gang' of toes clockwise and then anti-clockwise two / three times, whilst holding the foot steady with the right hand. This continues the toe-loosening and encourages increased circulation and removal of possible deposits resulting from loosening the metatarsophalangeal joints previously.

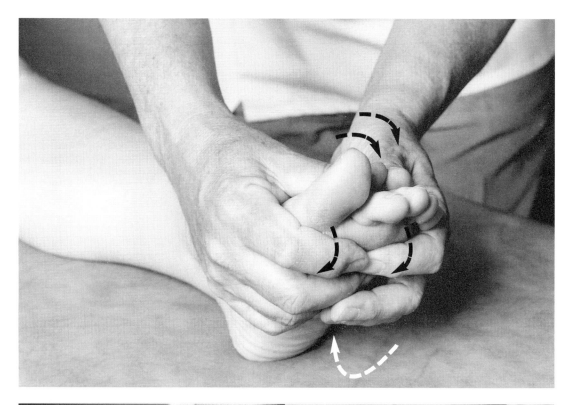

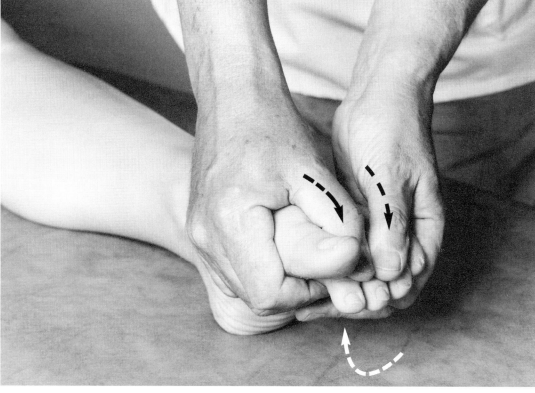

Figures 2/12 & 2/13: Loosening / Massaging Metatarsals and Small Toes.

Stand alongside the patient's leg and taking the foot in both hands, cup the foot as shown. Apply a sweep and bending of the toes downwards at the same time; the fingers under the foot pull upwards as the thumbs 'roll' over the toes.

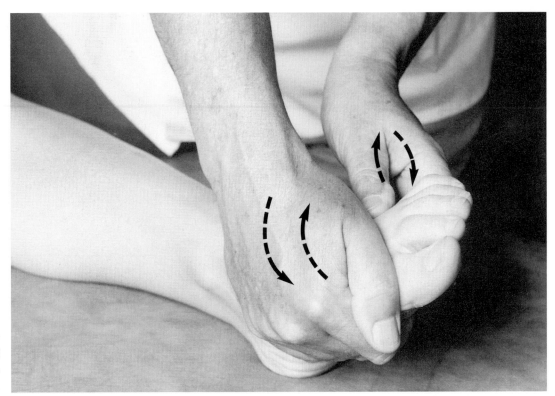

Figure 2/14:
'Shaking' and
Loosening the
Metatarsal Bones.

Remaining alongside the foot, hold it as shown and working across the foot use a combined bending / shaking (small vertical moves) to separate and loosen all the metatarsal bones.

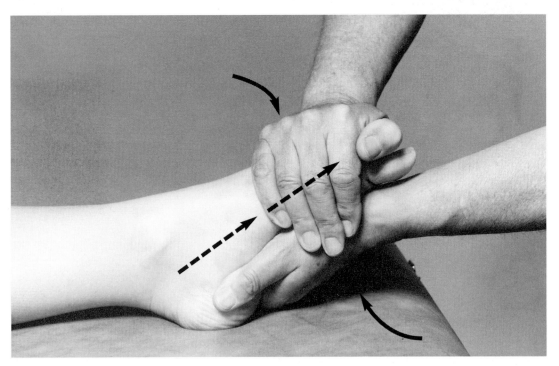

Figure 2/15:
Loosening / Releasing
the Fascia.

Left hand under and supporting the plantar surface of the foot place the right hand cupped over the dorsal surface. The foot is now the middle of the 'sandwich'. Moving across and then up and down the foot, making firm thrusts and slight plantar flexion, squeezing moves, to loosen the flesh of the foot.

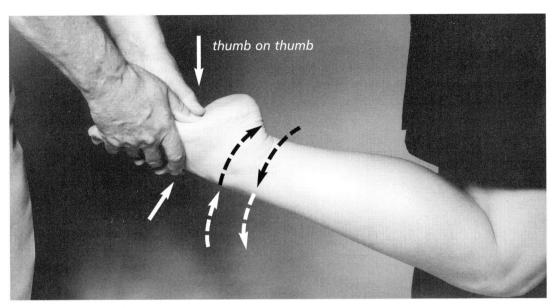

thumb on thumb

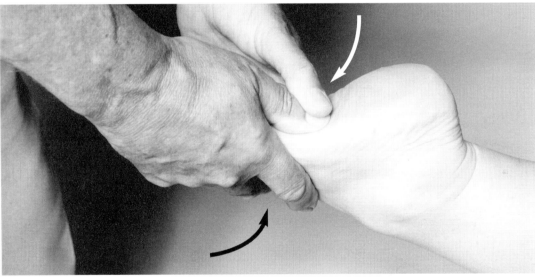

Figures 2/16 & 2/17: Cuboid 'Flick'.

This procedure is a stand-alone technique that is used only when a patient presents with pain under the foot (and sometimes referred pain in the lower back). Palpate the cuboid bone and assess degree of discomfort. If the bone is prominent, dropped downwards from the plantar surface of the foot and is painful, it needs popping back. The technique is not part of the routine foot and ankle loosening.

Ask your patient to raise their leg, as shown. Standing behind your patient, take the foot in both hands cupped around the foot and with the thumbs, one above the other, placed over the cuboid bone. Move the leg up and down until the patient is relaxed (and unsuspecting!). Check the thumbs are contacting the cuboid before throwing the foot upwards and bringing it down firmly and rapidly – pressing on the cuboid whilst flexing the foot with the inner edge of the forefingers simultaneously upwards – as indicated. There is a knack to getting this move correct, do not experiment. Compare mobility of the foot and ankle that has just been loosened with the one yet to be treated. Better still, ask your patient to compare and notice the difference by wiggling the feet and by taking a few steps. Then repeat the whole of the above procedures to loosen the hitherto untreated foot and ankle.

Part III – Revision of Reflexology Mobility / Relaxing Moves

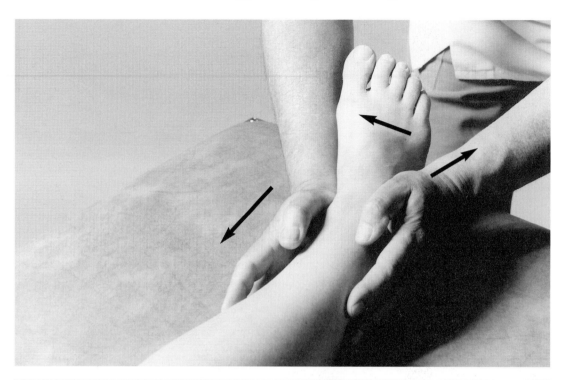

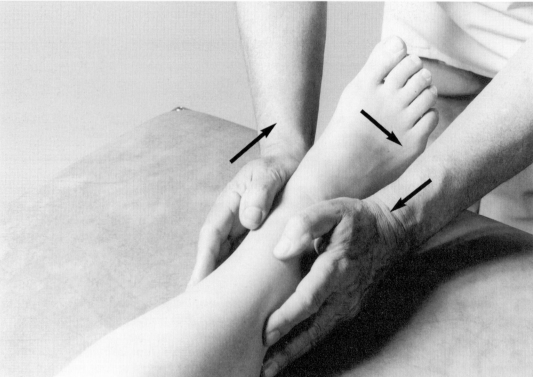

Figures 2/18 & 2/19:
Ankle Loosening.

Check that the pad of each hand rests naturally in the hollow just below the malleoli and then relax the hands before making the familiar moves to 'vibrate' the foot left and right, as the movement builds its own momentum.

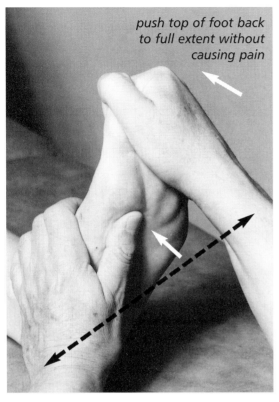

push top of foot back
to full extent without
causing pain

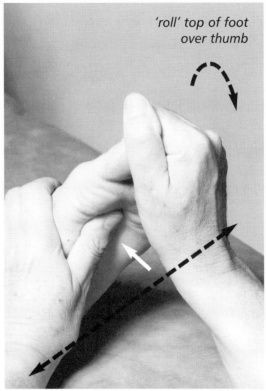

'roll' top of foot
over thumb

*Figures 2/20 & 2/21:
Diaphragm /
Metatarsal Loosening.*

Take care to move the top of the foot in extension before pulling it over the supporting 'peg' of the thumb (see Figure 2/20, above). The move is made across the foot, supporting each metatarsal head in turn and achieving maximum stretch of the upper part of the foot. The co-ordinated move should be rhythmical and pleasant for the patient.

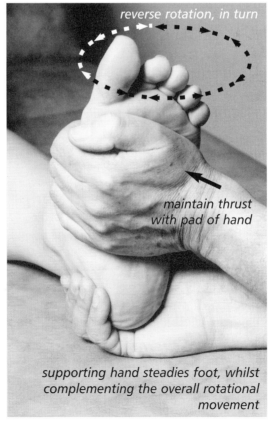

reverse rotation, in turn

maintain thrust
with pad of hand

Familiarity often results in forgetting to maintain the main thrust with the pad of the hand only (you can put a cigarette paper under the fingers and it should drop out). Maintaining thrust along the leg towards the patient, the foot is rotated, each way in turn, to loosen the foot and ankle.

supporting hand steadies foot, whilst
complementing the overall rotational
movement

*Figure 2/22:
Ankle Rotation.*

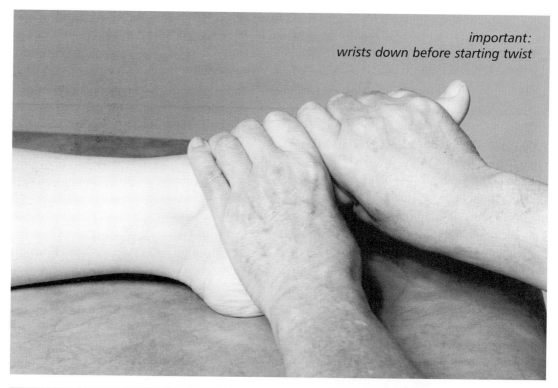

important:
wrists down before starting twist

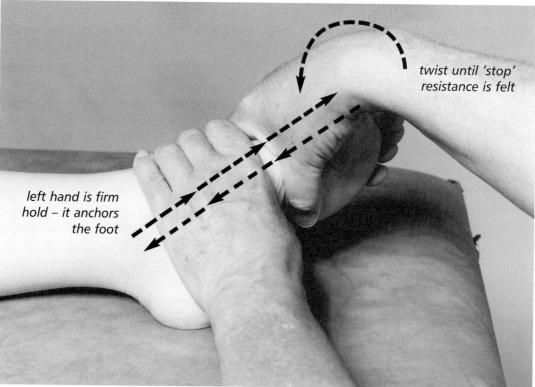

twist until 'stop'
resistance is felt

left hand is firm
hold – it anchors
the foot

Figures 2/23 & 2/24:
Spinal Twist.

Take particular care to drop the wrists before commencing the rotation that twists the spinal reflex. The foot is rotated until a definite 'stop' is felt. Lack of confidence can lead to the foot not being fully rotated with proportionate reduction in effect. Ensure each hand touches the other throughout and that the lower hand anchors as the upper hand twists, in a fluent, co-ordinated move up or down the foot.

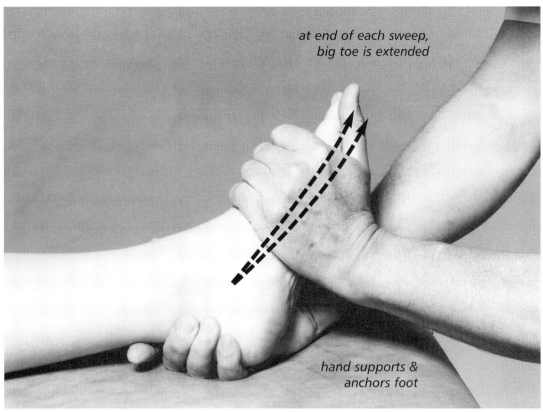

at end of each sweep,
big toe is extended

hand supports &
anchors foot

Figure 2/25: Spinal Sweep.

This move has proved to be relaxing, pleasant and of benefit to those suffering from back pain. The foot is anchored by the right hand, as shown. The left, starting from the lumbar reflex area – just in front of the medial malleolus – folds around the medial border and spinal reflex and 'sweeps' up the foot, using the outside plantar border of the hand to apply firm pressure, sufficient to extend the foot as the hand travels up the foot. At the big toe (hallux), it too is extended to complete the sweep which can be repeated five or six times on each foot per treatment; it is a reflexologist's version of spinal traction.

Faradic Footbaths

A very useful follow-on to the manual foot and ankle loosening moves is to use a Faradic Footbath. This uses two bowls of water with a faradic pad in each. The patient places one foot in each bowl and the electrical current is increased to a point where the muscles pulsate slightly. The duration of the bath is approximately ten minutes, depending upon the condition being treated. It is excellent as part of the treatment for flat feet and for dropped metatarsal arches.

If you do not have a Faradic Footbath, befriend a chiropodist (podiatrist) or a physiotherapist or refer your patient to one or the other in whom you have confidence in their professional ability.

Chapter 3

An Introduction to Dermatology

Introduction

Dermatology is the science that deals with the skin, its structure, functions, diseases and their treatment. The word is derived from the Greek '*derma*' meaning skin, and '*logos*' meaning discourse, so that a literal translation would be that dermatology is a 'discussion about skin'. The purpose of these notes is to acquaint reflexologists and similar therapists with the common skin disorders and their distinctive features. **This introduction should never be regarded as a replacement for the skill and judgement of a registered medical general practitioner, or specialist, to whom patients should be referred.**

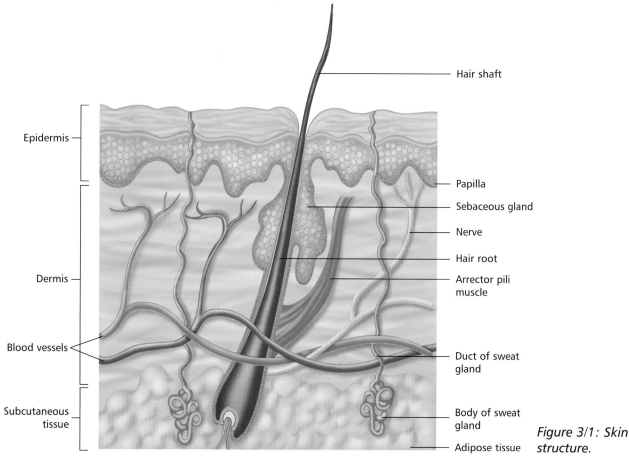

Epidermis

Dermis

Blood vessels

Subcutaneous tissue

Hair shaft

Papilla

Sebaceous gland

Nerve

Hair root

Arrector pili muscle

Duct of sweat gland

Body of sweat gland

Adipose tissue

Figure 3/1: Skin structure.

Skin Structure

The *epidermis* consists of a number of layers of closely packed cells (*see* Figure 3/1). Its thickness depends upon its location on the body and upon where exposure to friction is greatest.

The *dermis* lies between the epidermis and subcutaneous fatty tissue (see Figure 3/1). It supports the epidermis structurally and nutritionally and contains collagen (the protein that helps to hold cells and tissue together). The upper part of the dermis layer has elastic fibres within connective tissue; it also has nerve-endings that are sensitive to touch. The lower portion of the dermis contains hair follicles, nerves and the oil gland ducts of sweat glands and nerves that are sensitive to pressure.

Functions of Skin

- Regulation of body temperature.
- Protective outer layer; protecting the body from dehydration, bacteria and the effect of radiation and ultraviolet light.
- Receptacle of stimuli; via the skin's nerve endings that signal touch, pressure, pain and temperature.
- Excretion by perspiration that transports water, salts and organic compounds.
- Synthesis of vitamin D from sunlight. Substances within our skin convert vitamin D in sunlight into vitamin D_3 which becomes active in the kidneys.
- Water resistant.
- Production of melanin which gives skin colour and absorbs ultraviolet light.

Skin Conditions

The conditions likely to be encountered by a reflexologist, or similar therapist are:

- Acne vulgaris
- Dermatitis / Eczema
- Erythema
- Fungal infections
- Melanoma
- Psoriasis
- Urticaria

These will be dealt with alphabetically as a convenient reference instead of in order of commonality.

Acne Vulgaris

It is claimed that over 1.5 million people in the UK at any one time are receiving treatment for acne vulgaris.

Classification

There are three main categories:

1. **Mild Acne:** has small papules (nodules or bumps) and comedones (blackheads).
2. **Moderate Acne:** inflammatory lesions, some deep pustules and occasional scabbing.
3. **Severe Acne:** numerous inflammatory lesions, pustules, papules (small circumscribed elevations of skin), nodules and extensive scarring.

Within the above categories, there are five types of lesions:

1. **Open Comedones:** (blackheads) that are black in colour, and contain sebum and melanin which is a black pigment found in hair, skin and the outer membrane of the eye; they do not usually become inflamed.

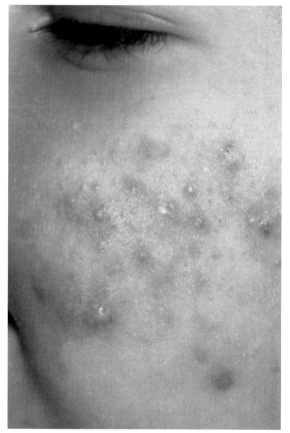

Figure 3/2: Acne.

2. **Closed Comedones:** (whiteheads) that are often inflamed.
3. **Papules:** small, inflamed, red lesions.
4. **Pustules:** which, as the name indicates, contain pus. They usually subside in 5 days – longer if they are deep.
5. **Nodules and / or Cysts:** are deep lesions, often painful and may take months to clear when scarring can be the residual outcome.

Cause
Over secretion (hypersecretion) of the sebaceous glands and inflammation of hair follicles that depend upon the presence of androgenic hormones. Hence acne is more prevalent at the time of adolescence. The pustules contain non-airborne bacteria that are not regarded as pathogenic (disease forming).

Location
Most common sites are face, back and / or chest.

Treatment
The aim is to prevent new lesions and scarring and to minimise the psychological embarrassment, depression, and lack of confidence that may accompany the condition. The Benzoyl group of creams, antibiotics and moisturisers are used, separately or in combination, for a minimum of 6 months. Removal of blackheads by using an extractor and ultra-violet β-radiation are other known treatments. Tea Tree soap has also been known to alleviate the condition.

Dermatitis / Eczema

The precise meaning of eczema is the subject of debate and generally the word is regarded as synonymous with dermatitis. The Greek derivation of eczema, 'ekzein' means 'to boil out', i.e. an eruption in the outer layer of skin. Similarly, dermatitis simply means skin inflammation. Hence the coincidence of these words in everyday medical use because they convey a condition involving inflammation and eruption of the skin. Inflammation of the skin can sometimes be due to an allergy but in many instances there is no known cause. Because many types of dermatitis are better known as eczema these notes will focus upon that general term in an effort to minimise confusion. The main types of eczema are:

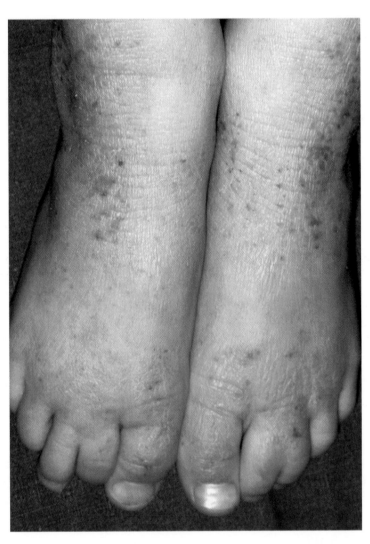

- Atopic
- Seborrhoeic
- Discoid
- Contact
- Venous (stasis)
- Photo
- Nummular

Atopic Eczema

'Atopic' refers to asthma, hayfever and eczema so that people who have a tendency to these conditions may also suffer eczema. It is common in babies up to 18 months old. An extremely itchy rash occurs usually on the face and inner creases of the elbow, groin or knee. The skin scales in these areas and small red pimples may appear. Scratching causes these pimples to ooze and infection may occur often as a nappy rash.

Treatment
Petroleum jelly for mild cases which keeps the skin soft in the infected area.

Figure 3/3: Eczema.

For more persistent or severe conditions, corticosteroid drugs may be prescribed. Consequently, reflexologists would concentrate their treatment upon the areas that correspond to the endocrine system generally and upon the adrenal area in particular. Affected babies should not be allowed to get too hot, which aggravates the condition, and cotton clothing in direct contact with the skin is preferable to other materials. The condition clears spontaneously as a child grows older, although it may come and go for a few years. Most children grow out of this form of eczema by the time they reach puberty.

Seborrhoeic Eczema

This is a red, scaly, itchy, rash that develops on the face (usually), nose, eyebrows, scalp, groin, chest and back. On the scalp it can be a cause of dandruff in adults and 'cradle cap' in infants. The rash can develop at times of stress but its precise cause remains unknown.

Treatment
Corticosteroid drugs and drugs that kill micro-organisms can help. Medicated shampoo containing ketoconazole, salicylic acid, tar and sulphur or zinc can be used to treat the scalp.

Discoid Eczema

These are itchy, coin-shaped, lesions that can occur on the arms and legs, mainly, of middle-aged men. They can be crusted or vesicular (pimpled), can remain for several months and they may recur.

The cause is not known but stress is thought to be a contributory factor. Once again, reflexology treatment could be both appropriate and effective in alleviating this condition.

Treatment
Corticosteroid treatment with an appropriate antibiotic.

Contact Eczema

As the name implies, this is a rash resulting from contact with certain plants, detergents (including residue in washed clothes) nickel present in watch straps and bracelets, chemicals, e.g. rubber gloves and condoms, some cosmetics, some clothing materials (wool affects some people when worn next to the skin) and some medicated creams. In summary, it is an allergic reaction to any or some of these products when they come into contact with the skin. The rash varies depending upon the irritating contact and the person's degree of reaction. Generally, it is often itchy, becomes blistered and / or flakes and is distributed according to the particular body part that has been in contact with the offending substance.

Treatment
Following patch tests, avoid the antagonistic substance; meanwhile, a soothing cream will reduce the tendency to scratch. A homoeopathic 'graphite' cream can be used to sooth.

Venous Eczema (Stasis)

This form of eczema tends to affect people aged over 50 years and is more common in women than in men. The rash is of patches of chronic eczema on the lower limbs. Varicose veins are often evident and ulceration may occur. The rash is vivid and may be accompanied by oedema.

Treatment
Corticosteroid ointments may give temporary relief; particularly for those with varicose veins whose skin on the legs can be inflamed, discoloured and irritate. The aim is to prevent scratching the affected area. Cotton is preferred next to the skin, and irritant materials such as silk, wool or synthetic materials should be avoided.

Photo Eczema

Occurs with people of sensitive skin such that it reacts to light – bright sunlight. The most common form is a cluster of spots or blisters on any part of the body exposed to the sun. Often they burst and dry, to leave small, temporary areas of dry skin, like an old blister-site.

Nummular Eczema

Usually occurs in adults and is of unknown cause. It appears as circular, itchy, scaling patches anywhere on the skin and looks similar to tinea pedis (athlete's foot) from which it needs to be distinguished. The condition can prove resistant to the usual anti-inflammatory corticosteroid creams.

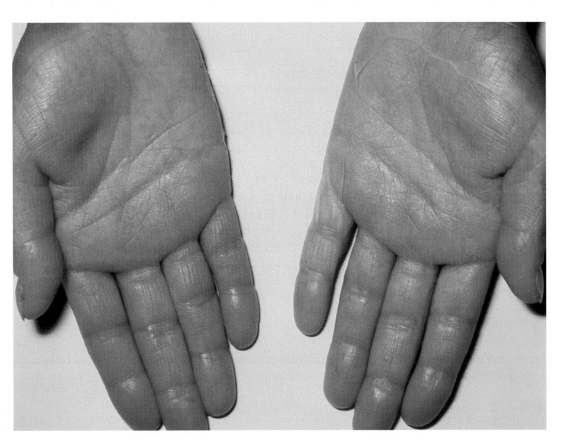

*Figure 3/4: Erythema
multiforme.*

Erythema

This is a general term from the Greek, meaning flush upon the skin. It is characterised by redness or irritation of the skin or mucous membranes caused by dilation and congestion of the superficial capillaries. Nervous blushes and mild sunburn are everyday examples. There are a number of skin disorders that feature skin redness, including:

• Erythema multiforme
• Erythema nodosum
• Erythema abigne

Erythema Multiforme

This is an acute skin inflammation that can sometimes affect the internal mucous membranes. It may be present in generalised illness.

Causes
Reaction to some drugs, such as penicillin, salicylate or barbiturates, or the condition may accompany a viral infection, e.g. herpes simplex (cold sores) or sore throats (streptococcal infections). The condition is most common in children and young women; vaccination reaction and radiotherapy are other possible causes.

Symptoms
Include red, frequently irritating spots; similar to measles rash. These spots may blister or become red, raised, pale-centred wheals, or 'target lesions'. Affected people may have fever, sore throat, headache and / or diarrhoea. Extreme form is called Stevens-Johnson syndrome in which the mucous membranes of the mouth, eyes and genitals become inflamed and ulcerated.

Treatment
This is for the primary illness that may be the cause of the erythema. If it is judged to be a reaction to a drug prescribed to overcome general illness, then that particular prescription is stopped. Corticosteroid drugs may be given to reduce irritation and inflammation. Those suffering from Stevens-Johnson syndrome are given painkillers (analgesic drugs), plenty of fluids (sometimes intravenously) and sedative drugs. The syndrome usually responds to this course of treatment but it is possible that the patient could become seriously ill as a consequence of shock, excessive inflammation or of inflammation spreading internally. **In summary, if a patient presents with a hitherto unknown itchy, red rash and is feeling unwell, refer to a registered medical practitioner immediately**.

Erythema Nodosum

This is an eruption of red-pimple swellings on the legs (shins usually) in association with another illness. Early lesions are bright red, raised and tender. The latter stages of the condition look similar to fading bruises. The condition is most common in the 20–50 years age group and affects more women than men.

Causes
Most common cause is a streptococcal infection (sore throat) but can be associated with other illnesses; tuberculosis and sarcoidosis. Can occur as a reaction to sulphonamide drugs.

Treatment
The treatment of the underlying condition clears the skin condition. Bed-rest and analgesic treatment assists and the condition usually responds and resolves within 3–4 weeks.

Erythema Abigne

This is red mottled skin that may be also dry and itchy as a reaction to overexposure to direct, strong, heat. Most common in elderly women and, in the days of the open coal fire, was quite common amongst those who habitually sat too close to the fire because it mottled the front of their lower legs. Can be eased by a soothing cream and by moving back from the fire!

Fungal Infections

Fungal conditions are quite common and caused mainly by two types of fungi; dermatophytes which grow in the outermost layer of the skin and give rise to tinea (ringworm) infection of the skin, nails and hair. The site familiar to most people for this type of infection is between the toes, in the soft interdigital skin and can also affect the toenails. The second main fungal type is candida albicans (yeast). This affects the skin and also the mucous membranes causing 'thrush'.

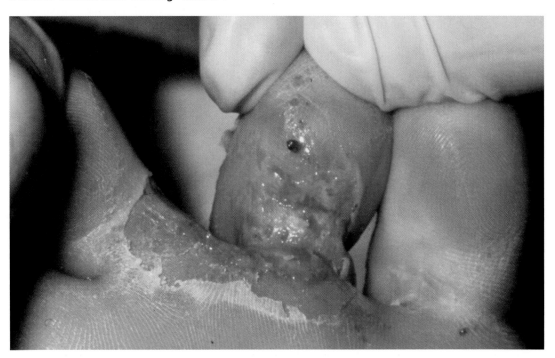

Figure 3/5: Fungal infections: tinea pedis.

Tinea Pedis ('athlete's foot')

This condition's common name has nothing to do with athletic prowess. The most likely locations where the infection can be picked up are in communal showers and changing rooms, hence its name. It thrives in warm moist conditions and, therefore, the site most commonly affected is between the spaces of the fourth and fifth toes where it causes irritation, maceration and scaling of the outer layer of skin. Infection can spread to the dorsal and plantar surfaces of the foot and into the nails where it starts as a yellowing of the distal margin and / or along the edge of a nail.

Treatment
This is by the application of proprietary creams such as 'Mycol', 'Daktarin' or Tea Tree ointment. This is followed by dusting the area with the powdered version of these products – taking care to 'dust' not 'clog' the skin. Regular change of footwear, general good hygiene and also dusting inside shoes and allowing them 'to air' when not being worn, all help to alleviate the condition.

An alternative and very effective treatment is to place the feet in a bowl of water to which is added a very small quantity of potassium permanganate crystals (available from most chemists) to create a pink solution. Hence its common name of 'pinky', by which it was known in the services. Soak the feet for ten minutes once or twice a week until the skin and / or condition clears. Allow the feet to dry in the air (to avoid cross-infection).

Tinea Unguium (nails)

This is the collective name of fungi that can infect the nail. Chiropodists refer to the condition as onychomycosis. The infected nails become quite brittle, opaque and brownish-grey in colour and finally develop a porous appearance. Infection starts usually at the distal edge of the nail and spreads gradually down and over the entire nail and the nail bed. This pattern of progress is accompanied by a gathering mass of debris under the nail which causes it to lift off the nail bed.

Treatment
Good foot hygiene is a prerequisite and often the initial treatment requires the attention of a qualified chiropodist. The nail is thinned to allow penetration of a topical antifungal preparation such as *onychocil* or *monophytol*. These preparations are painted onto the nail from a dropper bottle and should be repeated regularly for months until a healthy nail is seen to begin growing from the proximal root. **Intractable infections and onychomycosis associated with skin infection should be referred to the patient's general medical practitioner or, in the case of onychomycosis, to a qualified chiropodist.**

Tinea Corporis

This is a ringworm infection of the face, trunk or limbs. Erythema (reddening of the skin) and scaling recurs at the edges of plaques that may have pustules at their centre. The plaques spread slowly, healing at the centre, to give the characteristic 'ringworm' appearance. It can spread from an initial infection on the feet or in the groin and children can sometimes be infected from their pet animal.

Tinea Capitis

This affects the scalp and is found most commonly amongst school-aged children. It appears as generalised scaling of the scalp and / or as circular patches of hair loss. In severe cases, the hair loss can be permanent and can also affect the beard area in men. When inflammatory reaction is severe, the cause can originate from an animal.

Treatment
Often systemic anti-fungal drug therapy is required. Therefore, if the condition is reported by the patient or observed and suspected, **refer your patient to a general medical practitioner.**

Candidiasis

In its acute form, this condition often has a pustular appearance. A diagnostic symptom is the presence of small pustules scattered beyond the margin of main lesions. Candida albicans is a parasitic micro-organism of the digestive tract. However, a number of features increases the risk of this condition: poor hygiene, obesity, diabetes mellitus, warm, moist, skin-folds (under breasts and in groin), HIV, and an adverse reaction to some antibiotic treatments. Common types are:

Intertrigo. This affects the skin fold beneath the breast, abdominal creases, under the arms (axillae) and the groin. It is an inflamed area, often with macerated skin; sometimes creamy-white pustules are present. Also it can occur between the fingers which is where reflexologists may encounter the condition. Treatment is by anti-candida preparations and often combined with a hydrocortisone preparation.
Oral candidiasis. This is characterised by the appearance of white plaques on the mucous membranes. Can be caused by poor oral hygiene and from wearing dentures. Treated with oral anti-fungal preparations / lozenges.

Genital candidiasis. 'Thrush' usually takes the form of a sore, irritating, inflamed rash on the vulvae and / or entrance of the vagina (vulvovaginitis). White plaques are often visible and there can be a white vaginal discharge. It can be a distressing condition. Males may get similar symptoms on the penis. Treatment is by anti-fungal creams or systemic medication.

Melanoma

The Health Education Authority (1996) Information Sheet, entitled *'If you worship the sun don't sacrifice your skin'* stated there are over 4000 new cases of melanoma each year in the UK and over 1500 deaths resulting from melanoma. The number of new cases has more than doubled since 1974. It is vital that melanoma is identified and treated early because the prognosis is related to the depth of tumour when diagnosed. **Consequently, if there is the slightest suspicion by a qualified reflexologist, or similar therapist, that what a patient presents could be more sinister than a common 'mole', refer to a medical practitioner immediately. In short, if in doubt, refer**. But, for reference, there are various types of melanoma, of which the following form the majority:

1. Superficial Spreading Melanoma

This accounts for 50% of all known cases in the UK and can affect any age group, with women being at greater risk than men. This surface tumour spreads outwards and may contain variable amounts of pigmentation; its border is irregular.

If diagnosed and treated early it may affect the epidermis only. It can take from 6 months to 2 years for malignant melanomas to become invasive when a nodule may develop within it. This nodule indicates a deep dermal infection, with a corresponding poor prognosis.

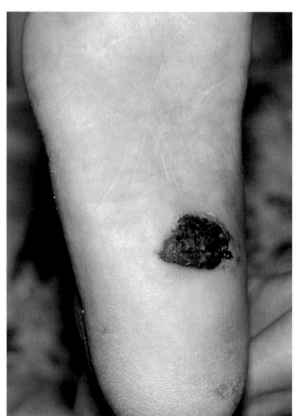

Usual sites for superficial melanoma are for women; arms and lower legs, face and upper back, and for men; trunk, face and upper back.

2. Nodular Melanoma

This accounts for 20–25% of cases in the UK and is more common in men than women. It is the most rapid growing and aggressive form of melanoma. The lesions are usually brown or black and instead of crusting, they are more likely to bleed or ooze – **which is a warning signal that should not be ignored**. These lesions may occur anywhere on the body.

3. Acral Lentiginous Melanoma

This is the least common in the UK, accounting for approximately 10% of the cases recorded. It may be seen on the palms of the hands or soles of the feet and can affect mucous membranes. This type of melanoma is extremely

*Figure 3/6:
Melanoma.*

invasive and can often be diagnosed too late. **It is vital that any pigmented lesions in the areas mentioned are investigated promptly. To delay could have serious consequences**.

Causes
The true causes are not known. They are most common in middle-aged and elderly people of pale skin who have been exposed to prolonged periods of sunlight. The increase in the incidence of reported skin cancer may be related to the increased affordability and availability of holidays by those in the Northern Hemisphere to countries that have long uninterrupted spells of bright, very warm, sunshine.

Symptoms and Signs
The tumour develops usually on areas of skin exposed to sunlight, but may occur anywhere on the body, including under the nails or in the eye. Usually, it grows from an existing mole which may enlarge to a diameter greater than 6mm, become lumpy, bleed, ooze, change colour, develop a spreading black edge, form a scab and / or begin to itch.

Treatment
Early diagnosis is essential because the tumour is highly malignant and can spread to other parts of the body. Diagnosis is by skin biopsy and treatment of a confirmed malignant melanoma is by surgical excision. The lesion is removed with sufficient surrounding margin to ensure all possible infected cells have been removed.

Psoriasis

This is a chronic, non-infectious, inflammatory skin condition affecting approximately 3% of the UK population. Of these people, about one third have a family history of the condition.

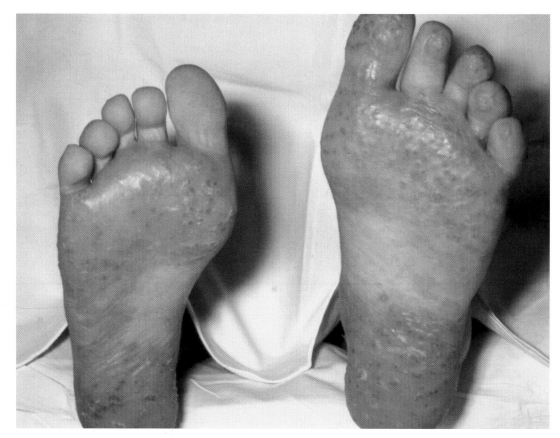

Figure 3/7: Psoriasis.

It is characterised by thickened patches of inflamed, red skin, frequently covered by silvery coloured scales.

Types and Sites of Psoriasis
Scaly plaques (erythematous) appear on the elbows, knees, lower back and scalp. They are extremely painful.

1. **Scalp.** Thick scale and redness at hairline and behind the ears;
2. **Nails.** Separation of the nail from the nail bed is common;
3. **Pustular.** Pustules on the palms of the hands and plantar feet.

Erythrodermic psoriasis is characterised by scaling and general pustules. The skin feels uncomfortably hot and there is overall fatigue, dehydration, loss of thermoregulation and the chance of heart failure.

Flexural (inverse) psoriasis occurs at "flexures" under the breasts, in the groove of the groin, and inside the bend of the knees or elbows. Common in women and the elderly.

Napkin psoriasis spreads beyond the nappy but can be cleared quickly. Can indicate a risk of developing 'ordinary' psoriasis in later life.

Urticaria

This term means the development of transient pruritic wheals. Individual lesions may be papules, arcs or plaques. They rarely last longer than approximately half a day. It is also known as *nettle rash* or *hives*, the wheals are itchy, white or yellow lumps surrounded by an area of red inflammation. Wheals can be sufficiently large to merge; forming irregular, raised patches. The most common sites are the limbs and trunk but may appear anywhere on the body.

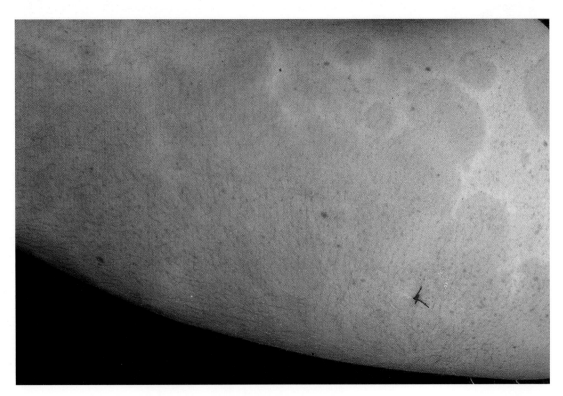

Figure 3/8: Urticaria.

Causes
Often not known but can be an allergic reaction in which histamine is released from skin cells causing fluid to leak from tiny blood vessels into the skin tissues. It may be caused by exposure to heat, cold or sunlight.

Treatment
Itching can be alleviated by calamine cream or by prescribed antihistamine drugs. Severe cases may require controlled drugs. Avoidance of aggravating factors helps.

Nail Conditions

See the tabulation (overleaf) and accompanying photographs for a summary of some of the conditions that may be encountered by reflexologists or practitioners of similar therapies.

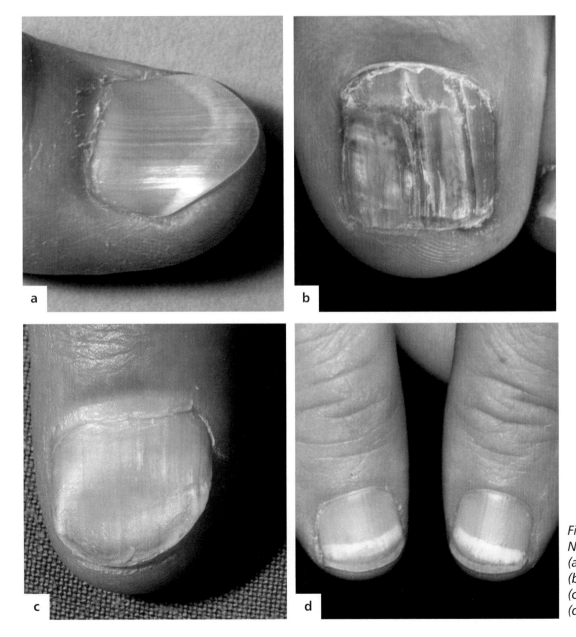

Figure 3/9:
Nail conditions,
(a) onycholysis;
(b) onychomycosis;
(c) koilonychia;
(d) beau's lines.

Condition	Possible Cause (Aetiology)
Abnormal Thickening (Onychauxis) from root to margin. Often accompanied by dark yellow / brown discolouration	Matrix damaged by: – trauma – neglect of trimming – fungi – systemic disturbance
Separation of Nail Plate from Matrix (Onycholysis) elderly most susceptible	Skin conditions, e.g. psoriasis, eczema; systemic condition/s or trauma
Retarded Nail-Growth (Onychatrophia) can lead to Onychomadesis	Debilitating illness; skin disease; old age; severe constitutional disorder
Splitting and / or Brittle Nails (Onychorrhexis) often with distinct longitudinal ridging	Can occur with ageing or result from constitutional disorder, e.g. anaemia, rheumatism. Can be due to malabsorption of vitamins and / or calcium, zinc or magnesium deficiency
Spooned Shaped Nail/s (Koilonychia)	Often **Diabetes Mellitus**. Also, can be due to debilitating deficiency such as anaemia
Transverse Ridges Across Width of Nail Plate (Beau's Lines)	Some past constitutional disorder causing temporary arrest of nail growth
White Spots on Nails	Can be from previous localised trauma or can be one sign of deficiency in zinc or vitamin A

Table 1: Nail conditions.

References

1. *Common Skin Conditions* (booklet). Nursing Times.
2. Levene, G. M., Calnan, C. D., White, G. M.: 2003. *Color Atlas of Dermatology*. Mosby, London. (ISBN: 0 7234 3298 8).
3. BMA *Complete Family Health Encyclopaedia*. 1990. Colour Library, UK. (ISBN: 1 85833 011 4).
4. Glanze, W.D. (ed.): 1998. Mosby's *Medical Nursing & Allied Health Dictionary*, 5th Edition. Mosby, London. (ISBN: 0 8151 4800 3).
5. Beaven, D. W. and Brooks, S. E.: 1984. *A Colour Atlas of the Nail in Clinical Diagnosis*. Mosby, London. (ISBN: 0 7234 0826 2).

Chapter 4

The Fuel – Aspects of Nutrition

Introduction

Much has been written already about nutrition and publicity given to various diets that claim to make us look like our idols. Given the stark choice of looking like some icon or enjoying good health and vitality, I guess most of us would choose the latter alternative.

If we regard our body as the earthly manifestation of "us" – our spirit – then it is our responsibility to take good care of it. This is not simply for personal benefit but to minimise the times we might otherwise bother others to care for us if and when we are ill.

However, many people in the Western world put 100% into their work leaving nothing for family, friends, interests and relaxation. It might be a cliché that we are what we eat but, like computers, if we put rubbish in, we get rubbish out. We need to put nutrition (body fuel) in and get only superfluous waste out.

Ideally, the food should be organically produced, fresh and full of vitamin and mineral nutrients. The air we breathe and the water we drink needs to be free of pollutants. Our thoughts need to be positive and our demeanor is best when it is relaxed and compassionate to the needs of others, i.e. free of stress.

Unfortunately, Western lifestyle has moved us in a direction that is opposite to these desirable, healthy aspects of life. We spend our day dashing about – mustn't waste a minute; live life in the now, in the fast lane of life's motorway. Eat a breakfast in the shortest possible time, grab a snack midday, eat on the run, attend endless meetings, balance budgets that some senior twit controls, write copious reports that get ignored, etc. Does any of this seem familiar?

We must make a conscious, almost continuous, effort to slow down, and get off the treadmill once in a while. So now we have to 'work' at relaxing! Health farms and leisure centres, with their workout areas have sprung up to encourage us to combine exercise with some form of relaxation.

One simple card we can all use is an 'ACE'. Not a playing card, but Vitamins A, C and E. vitamin A from carrots, spinach, brasicas, fruit; vitamin C from fresh fruit, salads, potatoes and parsley; and vitamin E from wholegrain, cereals, vegetable oil and nuts. Making sure these and other vitamins and minerals, either from fresh organic food or by supplementation, form part of our daily food intake, will help us towards maintaining good health and vitality.

In 2001 the World Health Organisation (WHO) declared that up to 70% of all cancers were related to diet. We need to be aware of the part free radicals and antioxidants can play in our effort to remain healthy and active.

Free Radicals and Antioxidants

To set the scene for consideration of what we mean by free radicals and antioxidants, we need to remind ourselves of a few basics.

An *atom* (from Greek *atomos*, meaning 'indivisible') is the smallest division of an element that retains the properties and characteristics of that element.

It consists of a core, or *nucleus*, that contains a number of *protons* (positive electrical charge) that are the same for each element; the total number is called the '*atomic number*' of the element. The other constituent is a number of *neutrons*; their number can be variable and when extremely disproportionate, the element becomes unstable. Spinning in orbit around the nucleus are *electrons* (negative electrical charge).

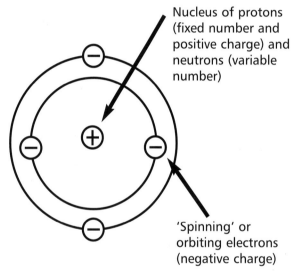

Nucleus of protons (fixed number and positive charge) and neutrons (variable number)

'Spinning' or orbiting electrons (negative charge)

Figure 4/1: Schematic diagram of an atom.

Two or more atoms constitute a *molecule* (from Latin *molecula*, meaning 'small mass').

A collection of molecules form an *element* (from Latin *elementum*, meaning 'first principle'). There are more than 100 of these primary substances that cannot be broken down chemically.

Two or more different elements bonded together chemically form a *compound* (from Latin *componere*, meaning 'to place together'). The elements combine in definite proportions and cannot be separated physically.

Note: An ion is an atom or molecule that possesses an electrical charge caused by a removed electron which creates an electrical imbalance.

A *free radical* is an atom or molecule that has one or more unpaired electrons in its outer orbit. Consequently, it becomes very reactive and unstable. An unpaired electron of either oxygen, nitrogen or carbon-based free radicals are of biological significance.

Free radicals are chemicals capable of independent existence; micro seconds in duration. They seek stability by attracting an electron from the outer layer of a neighbouring molecule to the 'unattached' electron to make a pair and to form a stable molecule.

The process of robbing a neighbouring atom or molecule of an electron from its outer layer causes a chain reaction between compounds, rather like a domino effect. One free radical can damage numerous molecules by this self-perpetuating process. This process of microscopic degradation is called *oxidation* that is a necessary process of decay in nature – from rusting nails to rancid butter to decaying animals (for which nature provides scavengers that feed off the carcass).

In humans oxidation by free radicals can seriously reduce the efficacy of our immune system and affect the rate at which we age. Heart and cardiovascular disease, cancer, auto-immune disease and skin disorders can be the consequence of unchecked free radicals at work. The process can be stopped by compounds called *'free radical scavengers'*. Most antioxidants are good free radical scavengers and one of the most significant is selenium, which is concentrated in the liver, kidneys and pancreas. It is yet another example of a little affecting a lot because there is less than 1mg of selenium in the body [1]. Studies have shown that the rise in 'modern' diseases like rheumatism, allergies, heart disease and cancer coincide with the decline of selenium in our diets. Could it be a root cause of late onset diabetes? Scope for research I suggest.

For easy reference at a glance, certain conditions have been highlighted in the following comments regarding vitamin deficiencies. These are the conditions that have been encountered frequently or which are a common cause of concern to patients seen in my practice over the years, whilst emphasising that reflexologists do **not** prescribe.

Some Vitamin Deficiencies

Vitamin 'A' Deficiency

Severe Deficiency: Burning, itching and inflamed eyelids; eyestrain; severe pain in eyeballs may be present; frequent sties; nervousness and exhaustion. Corneal ulcers are probable and mucus at corners of the eyes. Dry skin and rough skin often accompanied by irritation of whole body. Appearance of 'goose pimples' on elbows, knees, buttocks, and back of upper arm. Susceptibility to impetigo, carbuncles, boils and cysts in any part of the body. Hair dry and lack-lustre; dandruff. Profuse menstruation. Toe and finger nails ridged.

Mild Deficiency: Impaired vision; particularly noticeable whilst night-driving – the lights of on-coming vehicles destroy vitamin A in the eyes, clear vision is restored almost immediately after vehicle has passed. If vitamin A deficient, the driver is blinded temporarily – the length of time to recover vision being dependant upon the severity of the deficiency. Eye fatigue after watching television (irrespective of the quality of the programme!).

Foods Rich in Vitamin A: Kale, spinach, cabbage, lettuce, broccoli, carrots, apricots, tomatoes, peas, unbleached celery, asparagus, milk, liver, eggs, cheese. *Note*: It is necessary to have vitamin E with vitamin A, to prevent the destruction of vitamin A in the body.

Deficiency Disease: Xerophthalmia, night blindness.

Vitamin B_1 (Thiamine) Deficiency

Generally, this can be the cause of pain around the heart which, eventually, may enlarge sufficiently to be diagnosed as heart disease; shortness of breath on exertion; constipation; physical and mental fatigue; depression; sensitivity to noise; numbness in hands and feet; insomnia; neuritis in calves of legs.

Severe Deficiency: Leads to headaches, nausea and vomiting.

Foods Rich in Vitamin B_1: Wholemeal bread, brown rice, spaghetti, yoghurt and brewer's yeast. Vitamin B_1 is destroyed by heat and is inhibited by caffeine, alcohol and food-processing. The body does not store vitamin B_1 and excretes that which it does not need.

Deficiency Disease: Beriberi.

Vitamin B₂ (Riboflavin) Deficiency

With this condition, the lower lip may be crinkled and rough; flakes of skin peel off; corners of mouth split, crack, break open and bleed – becoming quite sore. These signs can come and go depending upon intake level of vitamin B₂. If chronic, crinkles appear radiating from the mouth and may extend upwards towards the nose.

Eyes sensitive to light. Night vision may be adequate but dim light or twilight presents difficulties. Person may become irritable and frustrated by dim light which is insufficient to allow them to work or to write; they need bright light. Eyes may water, lids may irritate, burn and feel gritty; consequent frequent wiping or rubbing of eyes that may become blood shot. High colour, broken veins over cheeks and under eyes.

Foods Rich in Vitamin B₂: Milk, liver, kidneys, yeast, cheese, leafy green vegetables, fish and eggs.

Deficiency Disease: Ariboflavinosis – mouth, lips, genitalia lesions (attachments).

Vitamin B₃ (Niacinamide) Deficiency

This can be a cause of diarrhoea in infants. In adults it can cause personality changes – those who were once positive become cowardly, depressed, apprehensive, suspicious and confused; they worry excessively and are moody, forgetful, uncooperative and emotionally unstable. They may have halitosis, sores, small mouth ulcers and their tongue is often coated.

They are tense, nervous, irritable, have insomnia, dizziness, recurring headaches and suffer from poor memory. Schizophrenics have been known to benefit from 1,000 to 3,000mg of niacinamide with each meal, combined with vitamin C and a high protein diet. Alcoholics also respond to this treatment.

Foods Rich in Vitamin B₃: Liver, lean meat, whole wheat, brewer's yeast, kidney, wheat germ, fish, eggs, roasted peanuts, poultry, avocados, dates, figs and prunes.

Deficiency Disease: Pellagra – general term embracing dermatitis, peripheral neuritis and changes in the spinal cord (that can lead to ataxia) anaemia and mental confusion.

Vitamin B₅ (Pantothenic Acid) Deficiency

This is a member of the B complex family and can be synthesised in the body by intestinal bacteria. Deficiency symptoms include fatigue, headaches, nausea, abdominal pain, numbness, tingling, muscle cramps and susceptibility to respiratory infections; severe deficiency may lead to peptic ulcer.

Foods Rich in Vitamin B₅: Meat, whole grains, wheat germ, bran, kidneys, liver, heart, green vegetables, brewer's yeast, nuts, chicken.

Vitamin B₆ (Pyridoxine) Deficiency

Can be a cause of depression, sore mouth, lips and tongue; insomnia, extreme weakness, nervousness, dizziness, foul smelling flatus, followed by a red, itching, rash around genitals. More noticeable sign is eczema often appearing first in the scalp and eyebrows and then around the nose and ears. Slight deficiency may cause anaemia and fatigue. Chronic migraine headaches often clear with supplementary vitamin B_6. Vitamin B_6, with magnesium, can help epileptics and 10mg of vitamin B_6 given daily has been claimed to overcome infant convulsions. 10mg daily may also stop or reduce nausea associated with pregnancy.

Foods Rich in Vitamin B_6: Brewer's yeast, wheat germ, liver, kidney, heart, cabbage, milk, eggs and beef.

Deficiency Disease: Anaemia, dermatitis, glossitis (inflammation of tongue).

Vitamin B_{12} (Cobalamin) Deficiency

This can be a cause of a sore mouth and tongue, nervousness, menstrual disturbances, unpleasant body odour, back pain and stiffness, difficulty in walking and shuffling gait. In time, the spinal cord degenerates and paralysis occurs.

Foods Rich in Vitamin B_{12}: Liver, beef, pork, eggs, milk, cheese, kidney.

Deficiency Disease: Pernicious anaemia, brain damage.

Vitamin C (Ascorbic Acid) Deficiency

Bleeding gums when cleaning teeth, bruising, brittle bones, pyorrhoea, possibly cataracts; vitamin C is necessary for the maintenance of healthy eyes and normal vision. Various infections leeches vitamin C from blood and urine, i.e. most illnesses deplete the healthy levels of vitamin C needed by the body which cannot store this vitamin.

Foods Rich in Vitamin C: Citrus fruits, berries, green leafy vegetables, cauliflower, potatoes and tomatoes.

Deficiency Disease: Scurvy.

Vitamin D (The 'Sunshine Vitamin') Deficiency

So called because we absorb vitamin D from the ultraviolet rays of sunlight. Deformity of head, chest and lower limbs. Menopausal women; hot flushes, night sweats, leg cramps and irritability, weakened bones, decaying teeth and irregular or protruding teeth (buck teeth), hair loss.

Foods Rich in Vitamin D: Fish oils; herring, salmon, tuna, sardines. Dairy products (note: some people now question the value of dairy products; others have benefited from reducing or avoiding dairy products completely. Care is needed, however, to ensure avoidance does not deplete the intake of vitamins necessary to maintain good health and vitality).

Deficiency Disease: Rickets, tooth decay, senile osteoporosis.

Signs of Rickets: Forehead huge, bulging chest caved in at top, with lower ribs flared outwards; legs bowed severely medially (causing knees to rub).

Infants (3–5 months) bulging forehead; in profile there is a straight line above the eyes of a normal, healthy child.

Other signs include narrow, under developed face and chest, buck teeth, irregular or crooked teeth, sloping or protruding chin and / or forehead, eyes very deep set.

Vitamin E (Tocopherol) Deficiency

Brown marks or spots on back of hands of middle aged or elderly people (also can be lack of sufficient selenium in diet). Muscular dystrophy – can be one cause of babies who are slow in their ability to sit up (i.e. at approximately 6 months old). Cross-eyes in children when due to weak muscles behind the eye. Similarly, bad posture of elderly – due to muscle-weakness. Hard scarring after surgery. Thyroid gland's inability to utilise iodine (vitamin E is vital for glandular function generally).

Foods Rich in Vitamin E: Wheat germ, soya beans, broccoli, sprouts, spinach, wholegrain cereals and wheat, eggs.

Deficiency Disease: Muscle degeneration, anaemia (low haemoglobin count) and reproductive disorders; destruction of red blood cells.

Folic Acid Deficiency

Anaemia, eczema, premature greying of hair, poor memory (might be due to hypothyroidism), lack of energy, anxiety, depression, tension, i.e. stressed condition generally.

Foods Rich in Folic Acid: Brasicas, wheatgerm, peanuts, sesame seed (also rich in zinc), walnuts, hazelnuts, apricots, melon, avocados.

Deficiency Disease: Anaemia.

Vitamin K (Menadione) Deficiency

Prone to bleed easily; haemorrhage (vitamin K controls blood clotting).

Foods Rich in Vitamin K: Brasicas, yoghurt, egg yolk, fish liver oil, watercress, tomatoes, potatoes.

Deficiency Disease: Coeliac disease, colitis.

Niacin (Nicotinic Acid) Deficiency

Tendency to headaches, intestinal gas, halitosis.

Foods Rich in Niacin: Lean meat, liver, brewer's yeast, kidney, wheat germ, eggs, poultry, avocados, dates, figs and prunes.

Deficiency Disease: Pellagra, rough skin, scaly dermatitis, 'black tongue disease', or deep red with fissures. Most commonly seen with those whose diet consists mainly of maize.

Minerals

Because minerals are inorganic they cannot be built within our bodies from raw materials, unlike protein, for example. Instead, we get them whole from the food we eat. Consequently, the quality of these minerals and their quantity depends upon the quality of the soil. Plants draw their requisite minerals from the soil and animals eat those plants. We eat the plants and some of us eat some of the animals that feed off the plants; it is an essential interrelationship, (*see* Figure 4/2).

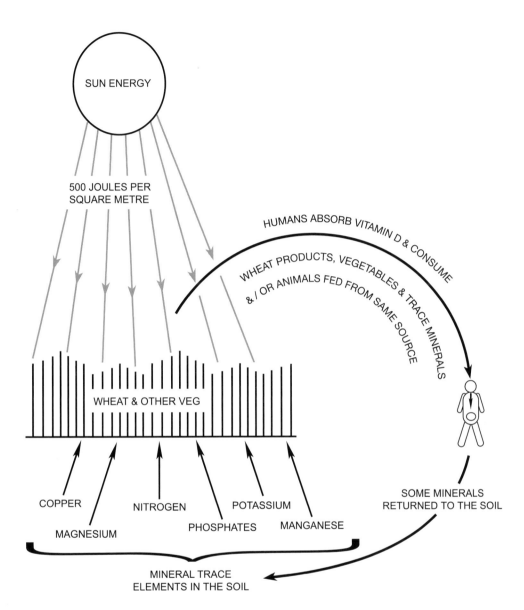

Figure 4/2: An environmental / food energy cycle.

In recent years, intensive farming practices and the widespread use of various pesticides has diminished the essential quality of the soil; it has caused an imbalance. Adding phosphorus, nitrogen and potassium can increase plant food production but can disrupt the balance between them and disrupts the ratio between them and other minerals and trace elements. A plant's ability to absorb the more sparse minerals diminishes as more fertilizer is added and the overall mineral content of a crop is chaotic. In addition, the acidity of the soil affects and limits the availability of absorbable minerals.

When we take account of all these factors, it is small wonder that we are no longer able to get all the minerals we need or get them in the correct balance needed to sustain good health from the food we eat. Hence the need to supplement our food intake.

Calcium Deficiency

Insomnia, nervousness, joint pain, high blood pressure, tooth decay, muscle cramps, osteoporosis.

Foods Rich in Calcium: Dairy products, green vegetables, soya beans, salmon, sardines, walnuts, parsley, prunes, pumpkin seeds. N.B. calcium, magnesium and vitamin D work together.

Deficiency Disease: Rickets, osteoporosis.

The ebb and flow of calcium in the body is influenced largely by two hormones; Calcitonin (CT) and Parathyroid Hormone (PTH). Calcitonin aids the depositing of calcium in bones whilst protecting soft tissue from an excessive uptake. The parathyroid hormone triggers the withdrawal of calcium from bones into the soft tissue on an as-and-when-needed basis. Once again balance is important. When the action of these hormones is in balance, all is well. This begs the question: Is the root cause of osteoporosis an imbalance between these hormones? It suggests that to say the bone porosity of the condition is due to a lack of sufficient calcium is an over simplification.

Chromium Deficiency

Dizziness, irritability after spells of no food intake; excessive sleep or drowsiness during the day, addiction to sweet foods, excessive thirst, cold hands.

Foods Rich in Chromium: Meat, chicken, shellfish, brewer's yeast, wholemeal bread, oysters, potatoes, eggs, apples, parsnips.

Deficiency Disease: Believed to be associated with diabetes and a possible factor in arteriosclerosis, heart disease and poor eyesight.

In the West – particularly North America and Europe – the high consumption of processed and refined food is thought to be a significant contributing factor in the increasing incidence of diabetes and heart disease due to the reduced intake of chromium (the hormone-accelerated growth of tasteless chicken is an example of processed and refined food). Brewer's yeast is by far the richest source of chromium which must be music to the ears of the fans of real ale.

Chromium is a vital factor in the formation of Glucose Tolerance Factor (GTF) that helps insulin to regulate blood sugar and it helps to regulate the metabolism of cholesterol.

Copper Deficiency

Copper improves the body's ability to convert iron into haemoglobin. A copper deficiency can contribute to poor thyroid function and is needed to make the amino acid Tyrosine (Tyr) usable. Also, poor pigmentation of hair and skin, and low energy.

Foods Rich in Copper: Beans, peas, wholewheat, seafood, prunes, liver.

Deficiency Disease: Anaemia, oedema.

Note: Copper is essential for the body's use of vitamin C.

About 30% of the copper we consume is absorbed by the stomach and the upper end of the small intestine (the duodenum and jejunum). Approximately a third is contained in the liver and brain and a third in the muscles. The remaining 3% or so circulates in the blood and soft tissue of the body. Copper is an essential factor in the production of a number of enzymes that are triggers for some vital chemical reactions; for example, the production of red blood cells in bone marrow.

There have been reports of patients tested and found not to have an iron deficiency, yet they continued to display the symptoms of anaemia, of pallor, lassitude and fidgeting. As a consequence, some of these patients' symptoms were diagnosed as neurosis – the "it's all in your mind" accusation. Yet in the 1980's research lead to the realisation that these same symptoms can be caused by copper deficiency. Pregnant and lactating women can be at risk because the foetus can take the mother's copper and, similarly, so can the breast-fed baby that builds its copper reserves during its first two to three months of life.

Iodine Deficiency

Weight gain due to poor metabolism, sluggish mental processes, poor memory, lack of energy.

Foods Rich in Iodine: Kelp, green leaf vegetables (organic, i.e. grown in iodine-rich soil), onions, seafood generally.

Deficiency Disease: Goitre, hypothyroidism (clinical symptom is myxoedema).

Iodine can influence our basal metabolic rate, rate of growth, the health of our skin, energy-level and mental development and alertness; all via the linked working of the hypothalamus and the thyroid gland. The latter holds about half of the 40mg of iodine used in the body; the thyroid needs iodine to form and secrete the hormones *thyroxin* and *triiodothyronine*. Lack of iodine causes the thyroid to swell when it is then called a goitre.

In the late 1980's researchers were concentrating on a group of substances called goitrogens, that prevent the thyroid gland from absorbing the essential quantity of iodine; one goitrogen they identified was the mineral manganese that is an antagonist to iodine. One of the richest sources of manganese is tea and another source is cabbage. School children now have a valid excuse to avoid cabbage at school meals. Nothing is that simple in maintaining good health, however, because cabbage is also a rich source of calcium needed for strong bones.

Iron Deficiency

Pale skin, fatigue and listlessness, poor appetite, nausea.

Foods Rich in Iron: Liver, kidney, heart, red meat, egg yolks, oysters, nuts, beans, pumpkin seeds, parsley, walnuts, dates.

Deficiency Disease: Iron-deficiency anaemia. Women more prone to deficiency than men (in one month they can lose twice as much as men).

Biologists consider iron to be the greatest influence in the body's fight to avoid anaemia, placing it in order of priority ahead of folic acid, Vitamins B_6 and B_{12} and copper. Deficiency in one, some, or all of which contributes to general anaemia.

Iron transports oxygen around the body in the haemoglobin content of our blood. It is this small amount of iron in blood that enables a low intensity magnetic field to help blood circulation and, in so doing, accelerate healing.

We each have about a level teaspoon of iron (3–4 grams) in our body. Haemoglobin, manufactured in the bone marrow, is responsible for the formation of red corpuscles. It is these red blood cells that carry oxygen from the lungs to all parts of the body. Half of the total iron content is taken up in forming the enzymes called *cytochromes* that enables the cells to utilise oxygen in their metabolic processes. Any remaining iron is stored in bone marrow, liver and spleen.

Magnesium Deficiency

Muscle tremors or spasms, muscle weakness, irregular heart beat, high blood pressure, constipation, tendency to hyperactivity and possible fits, lack of appetite (there can be other reasons), depression; magnesium is known as a stress-reducing mineral.

Foods Rich in Magnesium: Figs, lemons, wheat germ, brewer's yeast, grapefruit, apples, almonds, brazil nuts, beans, garlic, peas, raisins, cereals, grains, seafoods.

Deficiency Disease: Tremors.

Magnesium is a vital nutrient and a necessary part of our intake that ensures calcium is distributed and absorbed as, where and when needed in the body.

A healthy body contains approximately 30 grams of magnesium[1] most of it (about 21 grams) stored in the skeleton, the balance being held in the soft tissue.

Most of the magnesium intake is absorbed in the small intestine – another example for the need of healthy intestinal walls. Too much alcohol, sugar, and the use of diuretics can act against this process; and high blood pressure and hyperthyroidism can depress the amount of magnesium absorbed.

Tremors have been mentioned in the above quick-reference summary. The deficiency's effect upon our nervous system can span from a simple, but embarrassing, repetitive twitch of an eyelid to uncontrollable muscular tremors, over excitable behaviour and to convulsions.

Manganese Deficiency

Growing pains in children, poor sense of balance, joint pains, muscle twitches, convulsions.

Foods Rich in Manganese: Green leaf vegetables, raspberries, blackberries, grapes, strawberries, beetroot, celery, oats, wholegrain cereals, egg yolks.

Deficiency Disease: Ataxia (defective muscle control; irregular, jerky movements).

The majority of the body's manganese is stored in the bones, liver and kidneys. Its precise function and the amount needed for good health is somewhat vague in the existing literature. It is claimed, however, to play a part in energy production and is involved in the process of muscle contraction. I am familiar with a deficiency of magnesium and manganese leading to those annoying leg twitches that people sometimes experience, often in the evening when they have been sitting for a while.

However, manganese probably is known best for its part in the metabolism of carbohydrates. It helps the pancreas to store the sugar and starch absorbed from our food which, subsequently, is converted to energy.

Research has shown that when the pancreas is removed because of disease, the patient's level of manganese drops dramatically. Consequently, prescribed manganese often forms part of the treatment of diabetes and it might help in the creation of insulin. Conversely, it begs the question of whether there has been a gradual decline in the amount of manganese in the diet of Western people that might be contributing to the general increase in the incidence of diabetes – particularly late-onset diabetes.

Molybdenum Deficiency

Possible breathing difficulties and neurological disorders. Poor iron utilisation by the body, poor general wellbeing (although there are many other contributory factors to poor general health).

Foods Rich in Molybdenum: Dark leafed vegetables, wheat germ, lamb, pork, beans, lentils, tomatoes.

Deficiency Disease: No known specific disease.

Molybdenum is one of the trace elements and is concentrated mainly in the liver, adrenal glands, bones and skin. It has a part in the creation of enzymes that act as catalysts to fat metabolism. It needs to be in balance with copper with which it competes for a share of the body's enzymes.

Phosphorus Deficiency

Rickets, loss of appetite, general muscle weakness, osteomalacia (bone softening).

Foods Rich in Phosphorus: Almost all food contains some phosphorus; but of particular value are fish and poultry, eggs, nuts, whole grains and seeds.

Deficiency Disease: Rickets, pyrrhoea (pus from tooth area or socket), osteomalacia (softening of bone, with accompanying pain usually associated with vitamin D deficiency).

Phosphorus is essential for healthy bones; 80% of all the body's amount is contained there. It has an excellent bonding ability and is responsible for the laying down of calcium in the bones. The same property applies to the formation of a molecule vital to life itself, namely Adenosine Triphosphate (ATP) which supplies the body with all the energy it needs.

The body gets its energy from the digestion of fats, proteins and carbohydrates. These are absorbed via the gut as sugars, transported to cells and broken into minute particles called *mitochondria* to produce carbon dioxide and water. The energy released by this whole process is measured in calories and is the body's power source of life. The tissue cells subsequently excrete the carbon dioxide, together with urea – which is a continuous process-cycle at the cellular level.

Potassium Deficiency

Low blood pressure because of imbalance of sodium / potassium ratio (therefore, look to the area on the feet and hands that correspond to parathyroid, kidneys and adrenals), mental sluggishness and apathy, irritability, nausea, vomiting, diarrhoea, swollen abdomen, cellulite.

Foods Rich in Potassium: Watercress, citrus fruits, all green leafed vegetables, celery, parsley, courgettes, radishes, mushrooms, mint, bananas, potatoes.

Deficiency Disease: Oedema (swelling – fluid retention in tissues), hypoglycaemia (low blood sugar).

Potassium is concentrated in muscle tissue and is associated with enzymes that trigger muscle contraction; conversely, lack of this mineral leads to weakness and lack of muscle tone. Our levels of potassium decrease with age, hence the increasing frailty of the elderly. Perhaps its significant contribution, however, is the raising of the alkaline content of tissue cells. We know that a healthy body should be alkaline dominant and that a feature of every disease is acidity, so maintenance of the alkaline / acid balance is an essential feature of good health.

Causes of potassium loss include pre-menstrual tension, stress generally, oral contraception, heart malfunction and gastrointestinal disorders. Severe deficiency has been known to lead to erratic heart function.

Selenium Deficiency

Hardening of tissues, ageing. May be adverse effect on function of testes and the prostate gland in the male.

Foods Rich in Selenium: Bran, wheat germ, tomatoes, broccoli, onions, tuna fish.

Deficiency Disease: Premature ageing and loss of stamina.

One of the better known antioxidants and concentrated in the liver, kidneys and pancreas. It can help in the avoidance of high blood pressure and some of its consequences of heart attacks, strokes and associated kidney damage.

There are claims that selenium's ability to block free radical activity decreases the risk of cancer and some research has been carried out in China and New Zealand that supports this view. Both of these countries have soil that is low in selenium content. An American study showed that the incidence of cancer was nearly 20% lower in areas of high selenium[1].

Sodium Deficiency

Low blood pressure, rapid pulse, dizziness, muscle cramps, nausea, vomiting, heat exhaustion, possible head pains.

Foods Rich in Sodium: Salt (use sea salt rather than the common sodium chloride), carrots, beetroot, olives, shrimps, celery, cabbage, kidney, bacon, kidney beans, watercress, cottage cheese.

Deficiency Disease: Imbalance of potassium / sodium ratio that could affect normal growth; possible neuralgia.

We should not talk of sodium without also considering potassium because it would be misleading to think that the consequences of deficiency mentioned previously (*see* page 74), were because of a lack of potassium; it is due to the imbalance caused between these minerals. The healthy body maintains the balance between potassium and sodium or perhaps that should be said in reverse. The fact is there is interdependence one with the other. So a fall in potassium has a similar consequence as a rise in sodium to the point of exceeding potassium and distorting the balance between the two. This reminds me of a popular misconception regarding levels of sodium. Low blood pressure does not just depend upon reducing our consumption of sodium – particularly table salt. It is also dependent upon an increased intake of potassium and much more likely to be related to maintaining that vital and subtle sodium / potassium balance. Sea salt (rich in minerals) is preferable to common table salt that contains both sodium and chloride – hence its chemical name, sodium chloride.

Sulphur Deficiency

Dull, lank hair; brittle nails; fat intolerance (sulphur helps bile production by liver); poor skin condition (lack of tone).

Foods Rich in Sulphur: Beef (lean), fish, beans, eggs, cabbage.

Deficiency Disease: No known specific disease.

Sulphur is a constituent of vitamin B_1 (one of the vitamin B complex group), a number of essential amino acids and a constituent of keratin; the major component of hair, nails and skin.

It is necessary for the formation of collagen which helps to form bones, tendons and connective tissue.

Zinc Deficiency

Loss of appetite, poor sense of taste and smell, tendency to frequent infections and depression (could be cause and effect, i.e. if frequently ill, would be depressing in itself); white marks on more than two fingernails. Possible prostate problems.

Foods Rich in Zinc: Ginger, oysters, pumpkin seeds, beef steak, lamb, pork, wheat germ, eggs, peas, turnips, oats, almonds.

Zinc is associated with growth, sexual development and the maintenance of healthy, clear skin. Nutritionists, generally, recommend a daily intake, for men of mature years, say over fifty, of 15mg–20mg. Dr. Carl Pfeiffer of the Brain Bio Institute in Princetown, USA, estimated that an average 15mg of zinc is lost in a single ejaculation. So, to keep up with life's requirements, the daily intake is needed to avoid deficiency in zinc which is also believed to play a part in reducing the likelihood of prostate problems; particularly prostatitis (inflamed and swollen prostate gland). This is a condition that can affect adult males irrespective of age but most commonly occurring – if at all – in the upper age range. Typical symptoms are pain, difficulty urinating and loss of libido. The other condition (excluding cancer) is called *benign prostate hypertrophy* which is usually referred to as BPH. The name gives the clue; it is degeneration of the gland. It is estimated to affect 10% of men over 40 years and 80% of those over 80.

Dr. R. Bush of Chicago, USA, and Dr. Pfeiffer reported good results with doses of 50–150mg of zinc. Also, they discovered that this raised the male sperm count and increased the intensity of orgasms. Those wishing to conceive should not rush out and buy their beloved buckets full of zinc. It is not a sexual wonder drug and we must beware of increasing the level of zinc intake at the expense of copper and iron. Once again, balance is essential in all things and never attempt self-treatment without first consulting your medical physician.

This is not just a mineral for men. It is an essential component of ovaries as well as testes and can play a major part in the sexual performance of both genders. Even a minor deficiency of zinc has been shown to reduce libido. "Put zip in your life with a little zinc in your drink" might be an apt light-hearted slogan.

Other Beneficial Nutrients

Bioflavonoids

Helps strengthen capillaries and the healing of wounds and assists the effect of vitamin C.

Foods Rich in Bioflavonoids: Citrus fruit, cherries and berries.

Deficiency Disease: Signs are easy bruising, frequent sprains, varicose veins.

Inositol

This is needed for cell growth and is required by the brain, spinal cord (central nervous system) for the healthy formation and function of nerve sheath. It also reduces cholesterol and maintains healthy hair. It is essential for sugar and fat metabolism in the tissue cells of the body.

Foods Rich in Inositol: Eggs, fish, pulses, brewer's yeast, wheat germ, citrus fruits, nuts.

Deficiency Disease: Irritability, hyperactivity, insomnia and general nervousness can all be signs of insufficient intake of inositol.

Co-enzyme Q10 (Co-Q10)

If the body was an engine, this substance would be the spark plug. It is essential for health and wellbeing and is known also as '*ubiquinone*', from the Latin meaning '*everywhere*' which is an apt name because it is the energy spark of every cell in the body. It has a fat-like structure but acts as a vitamin. The heart and liver benefit particularly from an adequate supply of Co-Q10 which diminishes as we age. Primarily, it is sourced from meat and fish. In summary, Co-Q10 activates the production of body energy from food, whilst possessing powerful antioxidant properties and action.

This substance merits comment beyond those made for the other nutrients because of its important significance to our health. Research exists which demonstrates its efficacy regarding cardiovascular conditions.

People suffering from heart disease were shown to be deficient in Co-Q10. One 40-patient study involving severe heart malfunction, despite maximum medication, demonstrated improvement after taking Co-Q10. For 69% of them the improvement was significant.

Some patients who were awaiting surgery or transplants improved so much that they were able to come off the waiting list. Others made less dramatic improvement but, nevertheless, were able to walk, after being bedridden.

Supplements of Co-Q10 have been shown to be beneficial for those suffering heart failure, rheumatic heart disease, ischaemic heart disease (angina), irregular heart beat (arrhythmia).

Sports men and women have found that Co-Q10 improves their performance and stamina; intensive physical effort depletes muscles of Co-Q10. Somewhat similarly, regular supplementation of Co-Q10 can help those suffering from ME.

Co-Q10 is a safe supplement with no known case of overdose or adverse reaction with food or drugs. It is used widely in Japan and can help those with heart, circulatory problems, gum disease or loose teeth or those who push themselves to their physical limits.

Probably, this is a good point at which to draw breath and help you through the maze of balanced multi-vitamins and minerals on the market. On the following couple of pages are tabulations (as typical examples) from two very enthusiastic medical doctors; Dr. Rath[2] and Dr. Colgan[3]; Tables 2 and 3 respectively.

When studying these or any other combination, we need to understand the significance of the following terminology: *contents* must be listed on a label in order of weight; *active ingredients* are the potency or amount of each (not to be confused with contents) their effectiveness must have been proved in the laboratory; *sources* are the sources of the active ingredients, e.g. bovine organs; *bulk and excipients* are the 'make-weight' ingredients that may have specific nutritional significance. But for the significance to be claimed by the manufacturer or supplier, its effectiveness must have been proved in the laboratory.

The most effective products, therefore, are formulated to include primarily active ingredients and natural sources and to limit bulk and excipients; often the material used to form the capsule.

Enzymes

The food we eat cannot be utilised by our body unless it is prepared for absorption by enzymes. These are protein-based substances found in every cell of every living plant and animal, including us. They are an essential component formed from organic living matter; they are organic catalysts. They spark chemical reactions in the body that are essential for the efficient function of all our organs and glands and for the wellbeing of our overall body. They can be formed only from living matter and are not destroyed, being used over and over again with remarkable rapidity. All living matter contains enzymes. The body's chemical processes would not occur without the initiation of an enzyme acting as its catalyst.

Reflexologists will have met enzymes already – in their study of physiology and the digestive system. They can recall that protein is broken down into amino acids; complex carbohydrates into simple sugars (sucrose) and fat into fatty acids and glycerol. Every day the body produces approximately ten litres of digestive juices; from saliva, the stomach, liver, pancreas and intestinal wall – into the digestive tract. These juices contain hydrochloric acid (in the stomach) and the enzymes lipase, pepsin and renin.

Generally, oral enzymes have gained acceptance as valid treatment for a variety of digestive, gastrointestinal and pancreatic disorders. Research (most of which has been done in continental Europe with fewer studies in the USA and the UK), point to a positive role in the treatment of systemic disorders. Equally, lack of a vital enzyme can cause havoc if overlooked in the treatment of hypothyroidism. Whilst T_4 (tetraiodothyronine) loses an iodine molecule it needs particular liver enzymes in peripheral tissues to convert to T_3 (triiodothyronine) so that the body can utilise it; it is not sufficient for it to be swilling about in the blood.

Vitamins				
Vitamin C	600	–	3000	mg
Vitamin E (d-alpha-tocopherol)	130	–	600	iu
Beta-Carotene	1600	–	8000	iu
Vitamin B_1 (thiamine)	5	–	40	mg
Vitamin B_2 (riboflavin)	5	–	40	mg
Vitamin B_3 (nicotinate)	45	–	200	mg
Vitamin B_5 (pantothenate)	40	–	200	mg
Vitamin B_6 (pyridoxine)	10	–	50	mg
Vitamin B_{12} (cyanocobalamin)	20	–	100	mcg (*also* μg)
Vitamin D_3	100	–	600	iu
Folic Acid	90	–	400	mcg
Biotin	60	–	300	mcg
Minerals				
Calcium	30	–	150	mg
Magnesium	40	–	200	mg
Potassium	20	–	90	mg
Phosphate	10	–	60	mg
Trace Elements				
Zinc	5	–	30	mg
Manganese	1	–	6	mg
Copper	300	–	2000	mcg
Selenium	20	–	100	mcg
Chromium	10	–	50	mcg
Molybdenum	4	–	20	mcg
Other Important Nutrients				
L-proline	100	–	500	mg
L-lysine	100	–	500	mg
L-carnitine	30	–	150	mg
L-arginine	40	–	150	mg
L-cysteine	30	–	150	mg
Inositol	30	–	150	mg
Co-enzyme Q-10	5	–	30	mg
Pycnogenol	5	–	30	mg
Bioflavonoids	100	–	450	mg

Table 2: Basic cellular medicine programme. Source: Dr. Mattias Rath, M.D.

Fat Soluble Vitamins

Beta-carotene	12500iu	A (retinol)	7500iu
D_3 (Cholecalciferol)	400iu	E (d-alpha-tocopherol)	400iu
K (Phylloquinone)	75mcg		

Water Soluble Vitamins

B_1 (thiamin)	50mg	B_2 (riboflavin)	45mg
B_3 (niacin)	50mg	B_3 (niacinamide)	80mg
B_5 (pantothenic acid)	150mg	B_6 (pyridoxine)	50mg
B_{12} (cobalamin)	100mcg	Biotin	500mcg
Folic acid	400mcg	C (ascorbic acid)	250mg
C (calcium ascorbate)	250mg	C (ascorbyl palmitate)	150mg
C (magnesium ascorbate)	100mg		

Essential Fatty Acids

Linoleic acid	150mg	Alpha-linolenic acid	250mg
Gamma-linolenic	25mg		

Lipogenics

Phosphatidyl choline	200mg	Inositol	200mg

Accessory Nutrients

Co-enzyme Q-10	30mg	Citrus bioflavonoids	350mg
Para-amino-benzoic acid (PABA)	35mg		

Minerals*

Calcium (carbonate)	800mg	Magnesium (aspartate)	600mg
Potassium (aspartate)	100mg	Iron (picolinate)	10mg
Zinc (picolinate)	15mg	Manganese (gluconate)	5mg
Boron (aspartate)	3mg	Copper (gluconate)	500mcg
Chromium (picolinate)	200mcg	Iodine (potassium iodide)	100mcg
Molybdenum (trioxide)	60mcg	Selenium (selenomethionine)	200mcg

*Mineral amounts given are elemental (that is actual amounts of the element itself), not the amounts of the compound in which the element is provided. For example, calcium carbonate is only 40% calcium. So to provide 800mg of calcium, you require 2000mg of calcium carbonate.

Table 3: An example of a multi-vitamin / mineral programme. Source: Colgan Institute, San Diego, CA, USA.

If you are interested in learning more about thyroid-function and its widespread effect upon our health and general quality of life, I refer you to 'Hypothyroidism: The unsuspected illness' by Dr. Broda Barnes and Lawrence Galton, Harper & Row, 1976 (ISBN 0 690 01029 X) and to literature by Dr. Barry Durrant-Peatfield who had over 40 years experience of treating thyroid and adrenal dysfunctions successfully. Many of the patients I referred to him remain eternally grateful to him for improving their quality of life and, as a consequence, their happiness. Unfortunately, he has now retired from his practice but many of us owe him a great deal.

The best source of enzymes comes from uncooked or unprocessed fruit, vegetables and eggs, fish and meat. However, cooking and processing food destroys many, if not all, of its enzymes. Each enzyme acts upon a specific food and whilst they can act in a chain, one cannot substitute for the other. A deficiency or absence of a single enzyme can make the difference between health and varying degrees of sickness.

Enzymes with names that end in ' … ase' indicate the specific substance upon which they act. For example, phosphatase acts upon phosphorus, sucrase upon sucrose (sugar), etc.

In short, as long as our bodies receive or make enzymes, we live. Today, supplements of enzyme fortifiers have gained scientific credence and we are still learning about which foods contain what, what potency is needed for sustained good health, etc.

Most of the food we eat is cooked or is processed in some way and because the raw food we do eat (usually roots, fruit or nuts) contain only enough enzymes to process that particular food, our body must make most of the digestive enzymes mentioned earlier. This process can be reduced seriously by illness, injury, stress or ageing. Add to that the almost daily bombardment of pollutants and we can see the justification for helping the body with supplementation from a reputable supplier who backs their product-range with continual research and development.

From a treatment point of view, enzyme therapy falls into two broad categories; Digestive Enzyme Therapy (DET) and Systemic Enzyme Therapy (SET) both of which are self-explanatory.

It highlights the need to recognise that buckets full of vitamins and minerals consumed without the body's ability to absorb and utilise them is useless. I strongly suspect that the published 'scientific' studies that claimed supplementation was, in effect, money down the drain, failed to take into account the significance of, and need for, enzymes.

Those same critics often repeat the 'mantra', to stay healthy, all we need is to eat a 'balanced' diet. This is both misguided and out-of-date.

Absorption of nutrients varies between individuals, largely because of the variance in the condition of the gut and its ability to absorb nutrients through its walls. Even when they are absorbed their usefulness is greatly handicapped unless they are integrated into the cellular processes by the combined action of the enzymes necessary to maintain good health. Studies have shown that enzyme deficiency is a feature of most chronic ailments.

Systemic enzymes have been shown to have significant healing properties. They have been used in European countries for decades. Unfortunately, until recently the quite extensive research into their efficacy has been published in non-English journals. But the good news is that this is changing to the point where the formulations of oral systemic enzymes used in Europe are now available in the UK and the USA.

Dr. Edward Howell[4] spent much of his professional life studying enzymes, particularly those contained in raw food. He believed that enzyme-deficiency was the root cause of many chronic health problems.

Oral systemic enzymes can shorten the time needed to recover from sports injuries and accelerate healing generally. If given before and after orthopaedic surgery it can reduce the risk of thrombosis and promote faster healing and shorten the hospital recovery time.

Also, I believe that if we utilised the additional healing power of low-level magnetism, acceleration could be increased and hospital stay shortened still further.

In research studies and in clinical practice over the last few decades, oral systemic enzymes have been shown to be effective anti-inflammatory and immune enhancing agents with wide ranging benefits; ranging from sports injuries to cancer. They are being used and researched in multiple sclerosis, juvenile diabetes, tinnitus and fibrocystic breast disease[5].

Herbs – Nature's Medicine

There are many books and pamphlets about herbs and their medicinal value written by specialists more qualified to comment than me.

Consequently, this section is a selection of those used most frequently. The bibliography at the end of this chapter will provide more detailed information for those who wish to acquire more knowledge.

It is wise to avoid the trap of appearing to be all things to all people. However, it provides a more caring attitude to our patients if we can acquire valuable reference material. Then we can inform, whilst avoiding prescribing, and they can exercise their free choice based upon the additional information provided.

Agnus Castus (also known as *Chaste Tree, Monk's Pepper* or *Vitex*)

Is known for its beneficial properties concerning pre-menstrual tension (PMT) and other female conditions, including infertility. I remember our daughter was having some difficulty conceiving and my wife suggested she took agnus castus. Within a short time she was pregnant – much to the amazement of her doctor who reckoned it was impossible. After her fourth child, he kept his doubts to himself. Thankfully, my wife didn't take it! Research has indicated that agnus castus fruit increases levels of progesterone in relation to oestrogen. Also, it can alleviate acne that is associated with the menstrual cycle or with puberty of both males or females.

Aloe Vera

Has achieved great prominence in recent years. The plant originates from Africa and its leaves are rich in amino acids, minerals, vitamins and trace elements. Such richness makes it comparable to the basic make-up of a multi supplement and it is hardly surprising, therefore, that numerous benefits are attributed to its regular consumption – including improved digestive function, antibacterial and antifungal properties and the possible stimulation of the immune system.

Its fleshy green leaves are long, with spiked edges. These are crushed to make a juice or a gel. The gel can alleviate sunburn. It is also available in tablet form.

Artichoke

Both the Jerusalem artichoke (a close relative of the sunflower) and the globe artichoke contain a polysaccharide called *inulin* which is a food reserve found in some plants. Whilst it is a word so like insulin it is quite different and is not utilised in the organism of humans.

Artichokes are a high-class Mediterranean vegetables. The globe variety is a thistle-like plant of the daisy family. It has anti-toxic properties capable of stimulating the liver function and lowering cholesterol and lipid levels in the blood.

Bilberry

A familiar plant that grows on heaths, open moors and in woodland. Both the berries and leaves are used. Dried berries have an anti-diarrhoeic property caused by the action of the blue pigment contained in the berries. If using bilberry juice, it is important that it is unsweetened. Similarly, for those with bowel dysfunction, care should be taken with bilberry wines because they often contain sugar.

However, if bilberries are eaten raw – when fully ripe in summer – they can have the opposite effect, i.e. as a laxative. Taking the unsweetened juice for several months can help protect us against eye-strain, particularly for people exposed to long periods of computer work, reading, writing, drawing or driving, i.e. fixed focused periods of time.

Dandelion

Needs no introduction; many of us in pursuit of a lawn of which we can feel proud have spent many hours removing or destroying the plant. It does, however, have medicinal value. The leaves can be included in a spring salad and its root can be chopped and ground into dandelion 'coffee'. The dandelion, like other medicinal plants, has more than one useful active ingredient. Dandelions contain vitamins – particularly vitamin C – which probably accounts for its reputation as a spring cleaner of the liver and of the digestive system. It also contains substances that act like enzymes in stimulating the function of the liver, kidneys and cell metabolism.

Devil's Claw

A South African plant (otherwise known as *cape grapple* plant) that grows profusely on the red sand in the steppes of Transvaal. Young shoots sprout after the first rains and lie along the ground. Its dried root can be used as a tea to treat gastro-intestinal problems and rheumatic conditions; it is a powerful anti-inflammatory analgesic. It was introduced into Europe by a German farmer named G.H. Mehnert (the German for Devil's Claw is *Teufelskralle*).

Echinacea

Is a member of the aster / daisy family. It originated in North America and is a popular garden plant that has become well-known as an immune system stimulant and sustainer. The roots and the whole herb are used and contained within it, is *echinacoside* (a cycoside with antibiotic properties), volatile oil, inulin, betaine and other beneficial properties. Its benefits to mankind are due to their combined and synergistic effect. Old wounds and ulcers respond well. Taken by mouth, either in tablet or liquid form, it enhances resistance to antigens and stimulates the vascular and lymphatic systems. It has shown the capability of improving the body's resistance to infection, particularly influenza and the common cold – especially when taken as soon as early symptoms appear. Equally, it is well-known for its effect on the skin when taken as a tincture or applied as a cream externally.

Feverfew

Another common garden plant, bushy and daisy-like flowers and a fairly pungent, pleasant, perfume. When taken daily, it provides protection against migraine headaches.

Garlic

This is a member of the lily family, as are onions, chives, leeks and shallots. It is between a kitchen herb and a medicine. A 1600 BC record shows that Egyptians working on the pyramids downed tools because their daily rations did not contain enough onion and garlic to keep them fit and strong. Not only that, but garlic kept dysentery at bay and this was common throughout the East in those days.

The major constituent of garlic is *allicin* which contains sulphur that is responsible for the characteristic smell of garlic. Garlic contains Vitamins A and B, nicotinamide and vitamin C, enzymes, choline, thiocyanic acid and iodine.

The medicinal role of garlic is one very much based upon the totality of these principle substances. Perhaps allicin is the most significant; when ingested, it enters our bloodstream and is transported to all parts of the body. It is eliminated via the lungs and skin; which is why the breath and any sweat have the characteristic pungent smell.

Garlic helps purify and cleanse the intestinal tract, arterial walls, lowers blood pressure and opposes the build up of cholesterol.

Ginger

This is good for sore throats and upset stomach and is a warming blood tonic that boosts circulation. It can relieve nausea and it has been known to overcome travel sickness.

Ginkgo Biloba

Had a tradition of being planted in the garden of Japanese temples before being introduced into Europe in about 1720. Now seen in UK gardens and city parks, it is a rare sight in the wild. Its two-lobed leaf is its distinguishing appearance and these are shed in the autumn. It has a reputation for assisting vasodilation. Consequently, it should not be taken by anyone who is on Warfarin, Heparin, Aspirin or any other prescribed medicinal blood-thinning agent.

Ginseng (*Panax Ginseng*)

A herb that originates from East Asia. Interestingly, the name *panax* derives from *panacea* – the Greek Goddess capable of '*healing all*'. The Chinese name *jin-tsan* means '*life of man*' because the roots are thought to look similar to human figures. It is a perennial plant that grows on mountain slopes. The Korean Ginseng lays claim to being a potent variety of this herb that contains 13 different ginsenosides. Collectively these are believed to increase energy, enhance mental and physical performance and reduce the effects of a stressful life-style.

Hawthorn (*Crataegus*)

Generally, the flowers of the hawthorn (a common sight in hedgerows) are used for medicinal purposes; the leaves are used also. The hybrid red-flowered hawthorn found in the garden is a variant imported from North America but it is not used medicinally. It is also widely used as a remedy for some heart conditions and should no longer be regarded as containing digitalis-type glycosides. Whilst this fact is established, it went through a phase when 'the experts' argued that hawthorn was ineffective. Today we know it to be a plant that can be used in the treatment of cardiovascular diseases, provided the sum of its constituents in its natural state are used.

Hops (*Humulus Lupulus*)

Most of us associate hops with the brewing of beers. They are the fruit of plants that thrive in alder-swamps and damp hedgerows. The medicine, however, is derived from cultivated plants that are numerous in parts of the UK. It has a calming effect and is particularly useful with sleep problems. Also, it is said to be an effective antidote to sexual excitement.

Horse Chestnut (*Aesculus Hippocastanum*)

Well known to all schoolboys, the horse chestnut forms a valuable remedy for conditions of the arterial and venous systems. They have to be prepared specifically to make a useful product. The sweet, edible, chestnut (*castanea vesca*) is not used medicinally but its leaves are used as an expectorant in bronchitis.

Ivy (*Hedera Helix*)

Needs no introduction as it is found as a climber against any wall or tree within its orbit. It has a long history as a medicinal plant, dating back to the time of the Romans. Today, it does not appear to enjoy wide acceptance although some proprietary whooping cough remedies are said to contain its constituents, namely saponins and glycosides.

Linseed

Comes from flax (*linum*) that provides the fibres to produce linen cloth. It is familiar as a farm crop and as a laxative that acts as bulk rather than as a purgative. Also, it can be taken as a tea.

The farm crop is familiar as a delightful field of pale blue flowers and it is the ripe seeds – no doubt energised by the sunlight – that is used medicinally. The seeds contain mucilage, oil and protein.

Crushed seeds are available from chemists and health food stores and these can be added to a breakfast cereal or stirred into a pure fruit juice – at least a tablespoon full at a time is needed to achieve the beneficial effects and it should be continued for months rather than weeks; often 2–3 days elapse before the initial benefit is felt – so don't panic!

Sometimes linseed tea is used, particularly for stomach conditions. The mucilage content has a beneficial affect when the tea is drunk on an empty stomach in the morning and / or before meals throughout the day.

Milk Thistle (*Silybum Marianum*)

Another familiar and common sight in hedgerows and fields. It comes from the Mediterranean and many horticulturists wish it had remained there. Sometimes this thistle is confused with the holy thistle but the milk thistle has a long history as a medicinal plant. Latterly, it has been realised that it can be one of the best remedies for liver complaints – particularly hepatitis. Also helps to detoxify the liver following alcohol intake.

Peppermint (*Mentha Piperita*)

Is well-known as a carminative (a substance that relieves flatulence and associated colic). Originating from Eastern Asia it needs to be moved on a regular basis to avoid deterioration of its medicinal properties and to avoid its leaves curling up; it otherwise looses its flavour and aroma. So care is needed to transplant it every two years to a new site; propagating it from some root runners. Its leaves, when picked fresh from the garden, make an aromatic tea of superior flavour to pre-packed, dry leaves.

The active constituents of peppermint include tannins and bitters and menthol oil, which has an anaesthetising effect. Menthol applied externally can relieve itching of the skin.

Sage (*Salvia Officinalis*)

This evergreen, aromatic sub-shrub is used as a culinary herb on rich meats as well as having the medicinal properties of relieving laryngitis (as a diluted gargling tincture) and reducing menopausal flushes and night sweats or sweaty hands and feet. In each application it is the leaves of the plant that are utilised.

Saw Palmetto

The stems of the leaves of this small palm tree, from the southern states of America, are saw-toothed and very sharp; hence the name, saw-toothed small palm. The berries were used as a medication by the early North American Indians who used to chew them. Today, saw palmetto tablets or capsules are used to maintain prostate function and to have a beneficial effect on male libido.

Senna (*Cassia*)

A shrub of two main varieties, one grown in India and the other in North Africa. Its active ingredients are anthraquinone glycosides, that act on the colon, mucilage and tartrates that, together, inhibit the absorption of gut fluid, thus enhancing a laxative action.

Senna leaves or pods should not be consumed during pregnancy because they cannot only stimulate the muscle contraction of the colon but also of the uterus. In addition, senna is for short-term, corrective use; it should not be taken as a long-term laxative.

St. John's Wort (*Hypericum Perforatum*)

St. John's Wort grows on sunny slopes and in dry grassland or at the edges of pine woods. It gets its name because it begins flowering at the time of the summer solstice – St. John's Tide at the end of June. Its golden flowers are amongst the most beautiful of wild flowers of Europe.

St. John's Wort acts via the nervous system as an anti-depressant and in the treatment of bedwetting – particularly of psychological origin.

The action of herbs often is gentle and this gets confused with ineffective, sometimes maybe a deliberate ploy by researchers funded by vast pharmaceutical conglomerates.

The purpose of herbal sleeping drugs is to assist relaxation by causing the anxieties and stresses of the day to recede. Any mental depression tends to recede simultaneously.

Stinging Nettle (*Urtica Dioica*)

These plants grow where we live – along fences and on waste ground. Consequently, they are known as ruderals – they like to grow near human habitations.

Formic acid is a major constituent but plants also contain histamine, chlorophyll, iron, plant enzymes and minerals. It is hardly surprising, therefore, that its collective properties help to relieve rheumatism and gout. Also, it is a diuretic when used over long periods of time. It is available as a commercial juice and, in this form, it has been known to reduce cardiac oedema and venous insufficiency.

Thyme (*Thymus Vulgaris*)

Known best as a kitchen herb grown in the garden and as an ingredient in thyme and parsley stuffing, it also possesses medicinal properties. For medicinal use, the wild variety found in France, Spain and Italy is better than the garden variety. It grows to a greater height and has a higher concentration of the medicinal volatile oil. It is listed in monastic records and is proof of its use at a time in history when health-giving remedies were practiced in monasteries – long before qualified physicians came on the scene.

Thyme contains thymol, tannin and bitters; in addition to the oil and other substances. Their combined effect is the capacity to disinfect and clear airways, to thin mucus and to relax bronchial tubes. In dried form it can be used as a tea or infusion and, as a syrup it can be taken by the teaspoonful to ease bronchitis or a spasmodic cough. Once again, it should not be taken without seeking the help and advice of a qualified physician.

Tormentil (*Potentilla Tormentilla*)

If for no other reason my sense of humour would compel its inclusion in this list ('aperitif') of herbs and their medicinal properties. Surely this one is the most appropriately named because one of its prime uses is to stop diarrhoea quickly. In fact this ability to end torment makes it useful in the treatment of a number of digestive conditions: Crohn's disease (because it helps heal intestinal lining); colitis; diverticulitis (because this condition can give bouts of quite violent and sudden diarrhoea); IBS (irritable bowel syndrome) which we know responds well to thorough reflexology treatments.

It is a common European plant equally at home in very wet high-level moorland and forests (where it grows as a small, compact, plant) or in the dry soil of pine woods where it grows taller, presumably searching for sunlight. The root is used in medicine and possesses tannic acid and other astringents. These properties not only combat diarrhoea but, as a tincture, also alleviate conditions affecting the mucous membranes of the mouth and throat.

Yarrow (*Achillea Millefolium*)

Common to dry grassland and the roadside, this plant has white or pink flowers arranged in umbrella-like clusters. It contains bitters, tannin and oil and can be distilled to produce a distinctive blue oil. It counteracts inflammation and fever, being regarded as a tonic. Taken together with other soothing herbs, it can sooth acidic stomachs, indigestion generally, certain food allergies, colic and bloating.

Bach Flower Remedies

Dr. Bach's quotation *"Health depends on being in harmony with our souls"* has a ring of relevance to our lives today. It might, perhaps, be written as *"Health depends upon maintaining the delicate balance between mind, body and spirit whilst living in harmony with nature"*. The similarity is linked by experience and spans over 60 years.

Dr. Edward Bach, M.B., B.S., M.R.C.S., L.R.C.P., D.P.H. (1886–1936) was a physician and homoeopath who had a philosophy of simplicity and enjoyed his garden at Mount Vernon in Oxfordshire.

Every so often life throws up a genius of his or her time, such as Hanneman or Tom Bowen and Dr. Bach seems to me to fall quite naturally into that category.

He believed that attitude of mind plays a vital part in our health and in the recovery process from illness. When he died in 1936 he had developed a complete system of 38 flower remedies – prepared from wild plants, bushes or trees. In sympathy with the philosophy of homoeopathy and naturopathy, they work by treating the whole person rather than the disease or its symptoms.

He divided the remedies into seven groups that represent the conflicts that can prevent us from being or becoming our true selves. They are:

1. Fear
2. Uncertainty
3. Loneliness
4. Despair or despondency
5. Insufficient interest in the present
6. Over sensitivity to ideas and influences
7. Over-care for the welfare of others

For a number of years now I have become increasingly aware of the impact of emotion upon our health, happiness and general wellbeing. When we appreciate how minute quantities of vitamin B_{12}, for example, can have a disproportionate and dramatic effect upon our health, then it is perfectly reasonable to see that emotional disturbance from an individual person's normality can just as easily affect their health. At the very least it can affect how we feel, see the day ahead, regard other people.

Bach flower remedies address these aspects of our general wellbeing. Their purpose is to support a person's fight against illness by tackling depression, trauma, anxiety and other emotional aspects that can impede our recovery to full health. Also, they can be used preventatively by alleviating stress and anxiety.

The remedies can be taken alone or in conjunction with medical or other treatment. They are not intended as a substitute for medication and if worried, or in any doubt, a qualified medical physician should be consulted.

They are safe, with no known unwanted side-effects and are non-addictive. Their action is gentle and can, therefore, be taken safely by all ages – from infants to the elderly and they can also benefit plants and animals.

Probably a remedy known to many of us is Rescue Remedy which is a combination of five of the remedies designed to help us cope with difficult or demanding situations – such as an examination, delivering a speech or taking a driving test. I have known it work extremely well in calming children or adults needing first aid treatment resulting from an accident.

These flower remedies work specifically on the emotional condition of the person and on an individual basis. So that someone with multiple sclerosis (MS) may receive a different remedy to another with the same clinical diagnosis. This would be because one person may be resigned to their condition whilst another may be angry and determined to fight it – so different, but appropriate remedies would be used in each case.

The effect would be not to suppress the resignation, or perhaps negative attitudes but rather to transform them into positive ones – stimulating the body and the mind's self-healing and freeing the constitution to concentrate on fighting disease and stress.

You do not have to have signs or symptoms of illness to benefit from the remedies. It is possible to allow negative thoughts and attitude to creep upon us in times of difficulty or worry; it is at such times that the remedies can redress the balance and thus avoid the discomfort and inconvenience of illness.

Both animals and babies have been known to benefit from the remedies which suggests that they do not rely upon a placebo effect – the usual charge of the cynics. So they can be tried initially or as a last resort. Some gardeners found that giving Rescue Remedy on re-potting plants, for example, helped those transplanted recently to flourish. Presumably, if the plants died, the gardener could always take it himself, to offset the disappointment!

Dr. Bach worked himself to a standstill and at the age of 31 (in 1917) suffered a life-threatening illness. It was thought that only his determination to complete his work enabled him to survive. He had an overriding and strong belief that following one's natural talent (true vocation) is essential to spiritual and physical health. During my years in practice, I too have been struck by the high proportion of people that work simply to survive as distinct from earning money by utilising natural talent. Often, they have been influenced by their parents' desire to see them succeed or to have a secure or 'proper' job, whatever that means. Usually it centres upon a fear of the unknown or unusual. Imagine, for example, a feisty, personable, young daughter who wants to pursue an acting career and the consequent reaction of a father who is a cautious bank manager or accountant – the very antipathy of risk-taking and adventure. I can only wonder to what extent taking a job to keep the peace may be a contributory cause of certain groups of illnesses. If we see illness as an imbalance, then any emotional tug-of-war could become the root of an imbalance.

Dr. Bach's philosophy was both simple and profound, based upon the spiritual nature and innate perfection of human beings; health and happiness are dependent upon our being in harmony with our own nature and doing the work for which we are most suited. The paradox is that reason can, and is sometimes encouraged by others, to override instinct. Dr. Bach expresses similar sentiments clearly, as in his following words:

> 'Disease is the reaction to interference. This is temporary failure and unhappiness and this occurs when we allow others to interfere with our purpose in life and implant in our minds doubt, fear or indifference.'

Just as he identified the seven major areas of conflict that can interfere with our health (see page 87), so he identified the stages of the healing process as Peace, Hope, Joy, Faith, Certainty, Wisdom, Love. The 38 remedies cover all aspects of human nature and all the negative states of mind that Dr. Bach discovered that can affect underlying illness. It is not intended to give a precis of these 38 remedies because, in doing so, vital words and phrases could be omitted that would distort the value of Dr. Bach's work. Instead, for those who wish to know more and maybe integrate the philosophy into their practice, the following books are relevant:

'Lazy Person's Guide to Emotional Healing – Using Flower Essences Successfully', Dr. Andrew Tresidder. Newleaf (ISBN 0 7171 2985 3).

'The Work of Dr. Edward Bach'. Wigmore Publications Ltd. (ISBN 0 946982 07 4). This book has a comprehensive list of books, videos and audio cassette tapes.

'The Bach Flower Remedies', Nora Weeks and Victoria Bullen. C.W. Daniel Company Ltd., 1964, revised 1998. UK (ISBN 0 85207 205 8).

Useful address: The Dr. Edward Bach Centre,
            Mount Vernon, Sotwell, Wallingford, Oxon, OX10 0PZ, UK.

Australian Bush Flower Remedies

It can be frustrating when we get an apparent lack of response from a patient or when reflexology treatments seem to reach a plateau. Often the patient returns months later with the same or similar imbalances presented earlier. It can require a shift in the patient's consciousness to achieve further progress.

Whatever our prime therapy, at some time we have had patients whose response to treatment is less than experience suggests it should be because of something within them or their life; something they are not admitting to us or to themselves; a suspected mental or emotional block that holds them back. We may suspect that the constitutional imbalances revealed are manifestations of something internal that needs releasing for our treatments to be as successful as our patient would wish.

This provides a good reason to explore the potential of the Australian Bush Flower Essences to create the conditions for the patient to make the required shift of consciousness – thus removing the block.

Resolving these various psychological aspects can make a significant difference to the outcome and this is where the flower essences of Bach (pronounced *"Batch"*) or the Australian Bush apply and can be a very useful adjunct to reflexology and other therapies.

The Australian Bush Flower Essences are a part of subtle energy medicine and a pioneer in researching their remedial qualities is Ian White who founded Australian Bush Flower Remedies and gives seminars worldwide, has written three books, numerous magazine articles and been broadcast on radio and on television.

Whilst we should be grateful to Ian White, I cannot help suspecting that the Aborigines had very similar knowledge passed down to them (but not written down) for hundreds of years. Surely their very survival must, in part, be because of their awareness and knowledge of the medicinal properties of the plants and flowers that surround them in their native home environment.

Australia claims to have the largest number of flowering plants and the oldest of their kind in the world, due to their incredible resilience often in the most inhospitable of environments. It is speculated that these properties are reflected in the flower essences which are known to add to the user's own strength of determination to survive and to flourish in the face of adversity.

To quote Ian White:

> *"The purpose of the Bush essences is that they assist in clearing the blocks that stop an individual getting in touch with their true or higher self ... their own intuitive part which knows their life purpose. After my patients have taken these essences, I have seen an obvious and powerful alignment of their personalities and when this happens, true wellbeing and harmony occurs"*.

You will notice the clear similarity with Dr. Bach's philosophy and with the benefits of balanced chakra-energy (*see* Chapter 5). How remarkable to think that these two pioneers came to such similar conclusions from different ends of the globe and in two different life spans.

Introducing the use of these Australian Bush Flower Essences into our practices, is perhaps done most easily by using combination essences – synergistic blends of selected single flowers chosen to help with a number of the more common (often stress-related) aspects. They are a very convenient way of using the flower essences. Typically, they address the following broad factors:

• Self-esteem, confidence, achievement of targets / life ambition;
• Dealing with anger, frustration, grief, depression;
• Recognition of past traumas and other resolutions;
• Relationship difficulties, issues of sexuality, being true to oneself …

Ref: *Enzyme Pro News* Vol. 3. Issues 8 & 9 (Sept / Oct 2001)

Further Reading
Books by Ian White: Bush Flower Essences, Bush Flower Guide, Bush Flower Healing.

All available from: Enzyme Process, UK (*see* Useful Addresses).

Tissue Salts

For the maintenance of good health the body needs a balanced intake of tissue salts. The 'balance' would be different for each one of us because of the variance in our constitutions, life styles and metabolic rate. Age differences would be another variable, so the type and concentration must remain with the nutritionist and is outside the domain of a reflexologist who can, nevertheless, refer a patient to a qualified nutritionist.

A summary of various salts, their function and the consequences of their deficiency is presented as Table 4 on page 91, strictly for reference purposes only.

Acid / Alkaline Balance

This is in summary only and presented as Table 5 for guidance and as a quick reference.

Tissue Salt	Function	Imbalance or Deficiency
Fluoride of lime (calc. fluor.)	Necessary for all body tissues.	**Can cause:** varicose veins, late shedding of milk teeth and slow development of secondary teeth, muscle tendon strain, carbuncles and cracked skin.
Phosphate of lime (calc. phos.)	Found in all body cells and fluids: an important element in gastric juices, bones and teeth.	**Can cause:** cold hands and feet, numbness, hydrocele, sore breasts and night sweats.
Sulphur of lime (calc. sulph.)	Constituent of all connective tissues in minute particles and in the cells of the liver.	**Can cause:** skin eruptions, deep abscesses or chronic ulcers.
Phosphate of iron (ferr. phos.)	Part of our blood and other body cells, except nerve cells.	**Can cause:** continuous diarrhoea or (paradoxically) constipation, nose bleeds and excessive menses.
Chloride of potash (kali. mar.)	Constituent of the lining under the surface of body cells.	**Can cause:** granulation of eyelids, eczema and warts.
Sulphate of potash (kali. sulph.)	Interacts with the cells that form skin and internal linings of organs.	**Can cause:** skin eruptions, yellow coating at back of the tongue, feelings of heaviness and pain in the limbs.
Potassium phosphate (kali. phos.)	In all body tissues – particularly nerve, brain and blood cells.	**Can cause:** impaired digestion of fat, poor memory, anxiety, insomnia and a faint, rapid pulse.
Phosphate of magnesia (mag. phos.)	Element of bones, teeth, brain, nerves, blood and muscle cells.	**Can cause:** cramps, neuralgia, shooting pains and colic.
Chloride of soda (nat. mur.)	Regulates the amount of moisture in the body and carries moisture to cells.	**Can cause:** craving for salt, hay fever and watery discharges from eyes and nose.
Phosphate of soda (nat. phos.)	Emulsifies fatty acids and keeps uric acid soluble in blood.	**Can cause:** jaundice, sour breath, an acid or coppery taste in the mouth.
Sulphate of soda (nat. sulph.)	Acts as a stimulant for natural secretions.	**Can cause:** low fevers, oedema, depression and gallbladder disorders.
Silicic acid (silicae)	Part of all connective tissue cells, including those of hair, nails and skin.	**Can cause:** poor memory, carbuncles, falling hair and ribbed, in-growing nails. (Whole grain products provide the normal needs for this tissue salt).

Table 4: Tissue salts and their function (compiled from 'The Vitamin Bible', see page 94).

Acid Foods Avoid These	Neutral Foods Eat These	Alkaline Foods Always Eat These
All antibiotics	Apples	Baking soda
All fried foods	Apricots	Blackberries
Artificial sweeteners	Bananas	Broccoli
Beef	Beans – fresh and dried	Cantaloupe
Beer	Blueberries	Cinnamon
Butter	Buckwheat	Diakon radish
Carob	Cauliflower	Endive
Casein	Carrots	Garlic
Cheese, incl. processed	Cherries	Grapefruit
Chicken	Dates	Honeydew
Cocoa, chocolate	Eggplant	Kale
Coffee	Eggs – chicken, duck	Kohlrabi
Corn	Figs	Lentils
Jam, jelly	Fish	Limes
Ice cream	Goat cheese	Mangos
Lard	Grapes	Mineral water
Lobster	Honey	Molasses
Mussels	Lemons	Mustard greens
Nuts	Lettuce	Nectarines
Oat bran	Maple syrup	Onions
Oils – hydrogenated	Milk – cows, goat	Papayas
Peas – green, snow	Oatmeal	Peppers
Pork	Organic olive oil	Poppy seeds
Rye	Organic flaxseed oil	Raspberries
Soya beans, soy milk	Oranges	Sea salt
Sugar	Peaches	Sea vegetables
Veal	Pears	Soy sauce
	Pineapple	Sweet potatoes
	Plums	Tangerines
	Pumpkin	Watermelon
	Raisins	Yams
	Rice – wild, brown	
	Strawberries	
	Turkey	

Table 5: Effects of common foods on the body's acid / alkaline balance. Source: Colgan Institute, San Diego, CA, USA.

Water – Nature's Cheapest 'Medicine'

Finally, we give a few notes that I found useful when informing patients, or in the course of a 'therapeutic discussion' with them.

Fluid Retention

Drinking enough water is the best treatment for fluid retention. When the body gets less water, it perceives this as a threat to survival and begins to hold on to every drop. Water is then stored in extra-cellular spaces (outside the cells). This shows up as swollen feet, legs and hands. In addition, the urine becomes concentrated which in itself, can act as an irritant and give rise to feeling the need to urinate.

Diuretics offer a temporary solution at best. They force out the stored water along with some essential nutrients. Again the body perceives a threat and will replace the lost water at the first opportunity. Thus, the condition quickly returns.

The best way to overcome the problem of water retention is to give your body what it needs – plenty of water. Only then will the stored water be released.

Constipation

Water can help relieve constipation. When the body gets too little water, it syphons what it needs from internal sources. The colon is one of the primary sources. Result? Constipation. When a person drinks enough water, normal bowel function usually returns.

Muscle Tone

Water helps to maintain proper muscle tone by giving muscles their natural ability to contract and by preventing dehydration. It also helps to prevent sagging skin that follows usually after weight loss – shrinking cells are bouyed up by water, which plumps the skin and leaves it clear, healthy and resilient.

Weight

Studies have shown that a decrease in water intake will cause fat deposits to increase, while an increase in water intake can actually reduce fat deposits. Water suppresses the appetite naturally and helps the body metabolise stored fat.

The kidneys cannot function properly without enough water. When they don't work to capacity, some of their load is dumped onto the liver. One of the liver's primary functions is to metabolise stored fat into usable energy for the body. But, if the liver has to do some of the kidney's work, it cannot operate at full throttle. As a result, it metabolises less fat, more fat remains stored in the body and the weight loss stops.

Water helps rid the body of waste. During weight loss, the body has a lot more waste to get rid of – all that metabolised fat must be shed. Again adequate water helps flush out the waste.

How Much Water is Necessary?

Take your body weight (in pounds), divide it by 2 to give you your individual water required per day, in fluid ounces.

There are 20 fluid ounces to the pint, so by dividing the above figure by 20, gives the pints per day required to achieve balanced function of your constitution. Remember this is the water requirement and excludes other fluids. Preferably, drink only filtered water.

When the body gets the water it needs to function optimally, its fluids are perfectly balanced. When this happens, you have reached the "breakthrough point" that achieves:

• Endocrine gland function improvement.
• Alleviation of fluid retention and stored water.
• Utilisation of fat as fuel because the liver is free to metabolise fat.
• Return of natural thirst levels.
• Loss of hunger (which can be almost overnight).

If you stop drinking water, your body fluids will be thrown out of balance again, and you may experience fluid retention, unexplained weight gain and loss of thirst. To remedy the situation go back to the 'formula' described above and recapture another "breakthrough". (Ref. Donald S. Roberston, M.D., M.Sc.).

Finally, Don't Forget

When working the spine area, the vertebrae associated directly with the digestive process are:

T4 & T5	gallbladder and liver affecting, particularly, fat intolerance / emulsification	"afternoon tea" (between 4pm & 5pm)
T6	stomach	"dinner" (between 6pm & 7pm)
T7	duodenum (and pancreas)	
T12	small intestine (absorption of nutrients)	"lunch" (between 12 noon & 2pm)
L1	large intestine (elimination of waste)	
L2	appendix and abdomen (small lubrication general toning)	

So if we are in the habit of having lunch between 12 noon and 2pm, afternoon tea between 4pm and 5pm and dinner between 6pm and 7pm, it is easy to remember the above relevant areas within a total treatment session.

References

1. Erdmann, Dr. R. & Jones, M.: 1988. *Minerals: The Metabolic Miracle Workers*. Ebury Press, UK. (ISBN: 0 7126 1842 2).
2. Rath, Dr., M.: 2000. *Why Animals Don't Get Heart Attacks: But People Do!* MR Publishing, Netherlands. (ISBN: 0 9679546 8 1).
3. Colgan, Dr. M.: *The New Nutrition: Medicine for the Millennium*. Apple Tree Publishing Co. Ltd., Canada. (ISBN: 0 9695272 4 1).
4. Howell, Dr. E.: 1995. *Enzyme Nutrition*: *The Food Enzyme Concept*. Avery Publishing Group, USA. (ISBN: 0 89529 221 1).
5. Seller, M.: *Therapeutic Properties of Systemic Oral Enzymes*. Positive Health Magazine, Issue 71, p.38–41, Dec. 2001.

Bibliography

Mindell, E.: 1999. *The Vitamin Bible*. Arlington Books, UK. (ISBN: 0 85140 672 6).
Holford, P.: 1998. *The Optimum Nutrition Bible*. Piatkus Books, UK. (ISBN: 0 7499 1855 1).
Webb, M. Firing on all Cylinders. *Healthy Eating Magazine*, March 2000.
Healthspan Ltd., St. Peter Port, Guernsey.
Enzyme Pro News, Vol 2, Issue 11, November 2000.
Nutri Newsletter, Enzymes – The Spark of Life. 19th Nov. 2001.

Chapter 5

Energy – From Seasons to Chakras and Meridians

Environmental Energy

We live within an energy system and we have an energy system – life force – within us. For perfect health and harmony each part must be in balance and the cumulative energies must be in balance. This seems to be impossible because of imbalances occurring all the time and all around us. In addition, we are too insignificant as individuals to affect universal energy during our short life span, so there is a continual ebb and flow.

I see energy fields, rather as clouds, at various levels. There is the environment in which we live; the seasons of the year; the climatic conditions of the area in which we live; the energy within the earth and air of our environment; the four aspects of energy within us – body, mind, spirit and emotion.

Reminding ourselves of one of the basic laws of physics (that energy cannot be created nor destroyed) means that these various 'clouds' of energy fluctuate in strength and with time. So that if part of the energy of our global system is highly concentrated in one place at one time and then released by a detonator, we get a huge explosion of energy in the form of air-blast and fire. However, this chapter is about subtle shifts of energy that fluctuate with time, climate and our individual emotional feelings and state of mind. They are, by nature, constantly changing and the achievement of balance within our local environment and within ourselves coincides with a healthy existence.

Imagine huge 'clouds' of energy – from the vastness of the universal energy of sun and planets to that of the energy of our globe – which is part atmosphere and part earth energy. Within these clouds exists the sub energy of the continent or country in which we live or visit; within that cloud exists the energy of the locality of our particular habitat; the building in which we live or work has an energy field and finally, at the imagined centre of these 'clouds' of energy we – in body, mind, spirit and emotion – live out our lives in relation to time.

It is probable that these various clouds of energy affect our health and the way we see and feel about ourselves and about life generally.

Seasonal Energy

I believe we have lost our connection with the seasonal rhythm of nature. Our ever faster, frantic, lifestyle with its competitiveness and stressful tension is in direct conflict with the more subtle, serene, seasonal changes.

Winter is for resting, recharging our energy batteries and for conserving energy ready to spring forward in the forthcoming year, as it lightens and dawns a new opportunity. It is one reason why we gain weight in winter – it is nature's defence against the threat of cold and (in a prehistoric, natural state) food shortage; it is why we have a tendency to slow down – we are supposed to do so naturally, as part of the energy conservation process. Yet we go headlong at the same pace of modern life. It is little wonder that this produces conflict, stress and a crop of ailments that keep doctor's busier than ever. We need to be aware of and observe nature's clues. For example, how birds, that have not migrated, fatten themselves and become less active during the winter months; how squirrels winter store food and go into hibernation; how hedgehogs hibernate and fish descend to deep water, to escape ice cold and go into a state of suspended animation. The only species that does not modify its behaviour is us!

Spring is the time of awakening – a bursting forth from the bonds of winter – an opening of flowers and leaves and a time of renewed vitality for us all. We are more inclined to optimism, in tune with the joyous songs of birds, the bright colour of the spring foliage and flowers. Everything is fresh and bright and clean – the time of year that represents a new awakening, a new beginning and new hope. You can almost feel the surge of energy along with the lengthening hours of daylight.

Summer is a time of growth – transposing the germination to fully grown flora. It is when we achieve, grow and spread to cover new ground, new opportunities, new experiences, that can ripen in the autumn of our lives.

Autumn is for taking stock, of shedding that which has served its purpose and for beginning to slow down in preparation for the recharging of our energy process.

Seasonal changes affect our emotions or mood. Have you noticed how our mood tends to be gloomy in winter, brighter in spring, busy in summer and more tranquil in autumn? Whilst this is a grossly simplified generalisation, there is, nevertheless, some element of truth in it. We have probably been aware of these changes in others whilst not being too keen to recognise it in ourselves! Similarly, pessimism often coincides with dull, wet or foggy weather. Whilst optimism is more likely when the weather is clear, bright and sunny (with low humidity). In short, we are more inclined to be bright when the weather is bright and vice versa.

Subtle Energy – The Chakras

Many of the complementary therapies work on and with the physical and physiological aspects of the body. However, health is concerned also with a balanced and subtle energy system. The etheric body is an energetic form that links with all aspects of the physical body.

To quote from Dr. Richard Gerber's book[1]:

> "In its total expression, the etheric body is an energetic form which underlies and energises all aspects of the physical body. A more complete understanding of how the etheric body interrelates with and affects disease expression in the physical body

will provide valuable information to a new breed of physicians who are attempting to evolve beyond traditional medical dogma in their attempts to create new and more effective approaches towards healing human illness. The medical establishment will benefit by beginning to learn the true underlying causes of health. The gradual acceptance of the new information will eventually foster the creation of an energy medicine approach to preventative medicine."

When we consider the body's energy there are various 'fields' or surrounding clouds of energy around the body in addition to the internal energy. The spectrum is from the energy of an individual tissue cell right up, or out, to the higher spiritual level.

We have our physical body where most of the time, effort and cost has been concentrated when restoring or maintaining health. Beyond is the etheric level, linked by the chakra nadis network. The additional links from the physical body of anatomy, physiological and nervous system is provided by the meridian system. Acupuncture, acupressure and the bioelectronic systems of therapy utilise these links.

The *nadis* are a network of subtle energy channels between the chakras and are interwoven with our physical nervous system. They can affect the quality of nerve transmission, particularly the network between the brain, spinal cord and the peripheral nerves. The esoteric 'layer' of energy, in turn, is enveloped (but not separated from) the astral 'cloud' of energy. It is as if we have shrouds of energy of which the esoteric is intermediate to the astral shroud. Conversely, their dysfunction can influence the pathological changes of the nervous system. We can only wonder to what extent these subtleties are taken into account when researching the causes and the subsequent treatment of motor neurone diseases.

Moving further outwards from the physical body brings us to the astral level, the mental level and to the higher, spiritual level. The fascinating thing is that some or all of these bioenergetic aspects have an affect upon our health and wellbeing (how we feel and how we perceive ourselves in relation to others and to our social and local environment).

These features of health, like the various medical procedures and like the numerous supporting therapies, together, are as tiles that abut and link to form the roof of total health care under which we could be protected.

Hitherto, chakras have been regarded as spinning vortexes of subtle energy. From the work and writing of Dr. Richard Gerber[1] we know that they act also as *transducers*, processing vibrational energy of particular frequencies.

A transducer, from physics, is a devise that converts a signal from one form of energy into another. It is similar to a radio receiver converting an electrical signal to sounds of voice or music.

The ability to detect and work with subtle energies is based upon this transducer system that involves our endocrine and nervous systems, together with our biofield to which these systems are connected (*see* Table 6). This master control system, in turn, is interactive with our hormone levels that affect our mood and our behaviour. If the chakras are out of balance it has an effect upon the entire network.

The chakras influence the flow, or balance, of higher or subtle energies associated with the etheric shroud of the physical body. In turn, this energy translates to the central and peripheral nervous system, hormonal balance and thence cellular changes throughout the body.

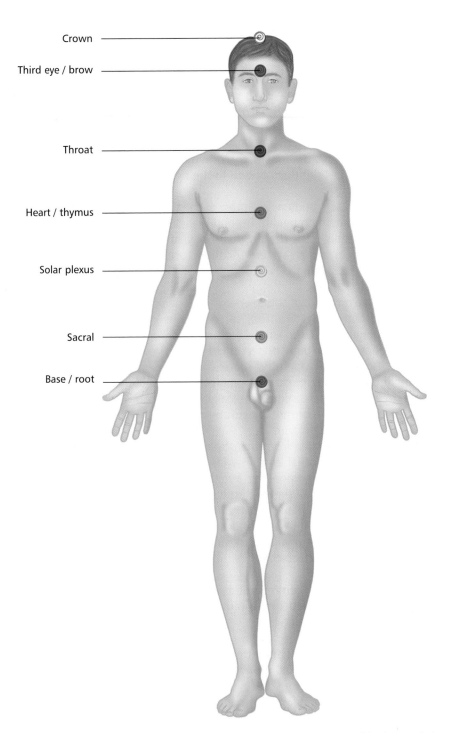

Crown

Third eye / brow

Throat

Heart / thymus

Solar plexus

Sacral

Base / root

Figure 5/1: The seven major chakras.

When we link this with the research of Dr. Candice Pert[2] concerning emotional balance, it is feasible to suggest that chakra balance, to an extent unknown or unproven, relates also to our emotional wellbeing. Dr. Pert showed that the transmission of signals was not confined to the nervous system but was inter-cellular. Each cell has the capability to 'talk to' its neighbour.

We can now see how the touch therapies, like reflexology, do indeed affect emotional wellbeing and are not necessarily confined to relaxing patients and to reducing the stress under which they are living. It is a reverse process; from physical (cell level) to etheric. I must stress that this is a personal hypothesis only. Maybe someone might like to test its validity; it promises to be an intriguing path of discovery.

The emergence of the discipline of psychoneuroimmunology is a more recent recognition of the interdependence between the energetic function of the brain, endocrine, immune and nervous systems.

I believe the greatest influence of the chakras is upon our emotions. In practice, it became more and more evident that the impact of emotional disturbance had a significant influence upon general health. Indeed, many believe that a serious breakdown of health can, in part at least, be attributed to a previous and serious emotional experience and simultaneous disturbance, often preceeding the onset of physical symptoms of ill health by up to two years.

The body has seven energy centres or vortexes that the Hindus call *chakras*. They are powerful electrical fields, invisible nerve centres, but none-the-less real. In Ayurvedic and in yogi theory these centres are aligned vertically up the centre of the body from the base of the pelvic girdle to the top of the head (*see* Figure 5/1).

Dr. Keith Scott-Mumby[3] writes that there are 360 known chakras of the body; numerically, almost one for every day of the year. For reflexologists, it is sufficient that there are seven major chakras and eight minor ones. The minor ones are in the palm of each hand, on the inside (crease) of each elbow, at each patella (knee) and at the anterior fold of each ankle joint.

The lowest, the *root* or *base*, chakra centres on the adrenal glands; the sixth (*sacral*) centres on the ovaries / testes; the fifth on the *solar plexus* of our nervous system and pancreas; the fourth (*heart / thymus*) chakra centres on the thymus gland at the mid sternum area; the third and second chakras centre on the thyroid and pituitary glands respectively and the uppermost, first (*crown*) chakra centres upon the pineal gland, posterior to and above it (*see* Tables 6 & 7 and Figures 5/3–5/5).

Chakras, ignored for so long by Western scientists and the medical profession, are now beginning to be recognised because subtle energy technologies have been developed that allow their existence to be verified. Just how this acceptance is integrated into our Western approach to health is a different matter. I can suggest only that we 'watch this space'; possibly an apt phrase in some circumstances.

Chapter 4 dealt with the various physical nutrients needed to promote and maintain healthy cellular growth at the molecular level and some of the consequences of depletion. In this chapter, we take 'nutrients' in a broader context where 'the food' is in the form of subtle energy. The subtle energy currents conveyed by the various chakras and along the meridians (energy routes) are necessary to maintain a healthy balance at the etheric level. Changes at this level precede those manifested at the physical level.

This energy is believed to enter the body via the crown chakra and to travel via the pineal gland and the pituitary gland of the endocrine system and the spinal cord linking, in turn, with the various nerve plexuses (*see* Figure 5/2).

Anatomically, each major chakra is associated with a major autonomic nerve plexus and with a respective endocrine gland, as summarised by Table 6. Figure 5/2 is a simplified representation of these nerve plexuses and their corresponding chakras.

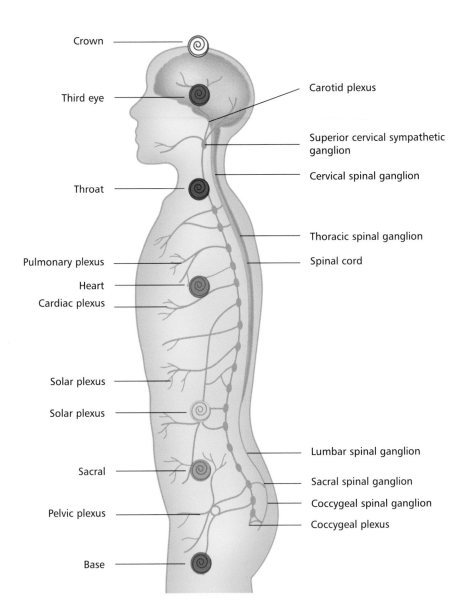

Figure 5/2: The seven major chakras and the associated nerve plexuses.

Chakras	Associated Endocrine Organs	Associated Area of Spine
1. Crown	Pineal	Cranium
2. Third eye	Pituitary	C1–C4
3. Throat	Thyroid	C5–T3
4. Heart	Thymus	T4–T8
5. Solar plexus	Pancreas	T9–L2
6. Sacral	Gonads	L3–S2
7. Base	Adrenals	S3–coccyx

Table 6: Association of main chakras to the endocrine system and to the spine.

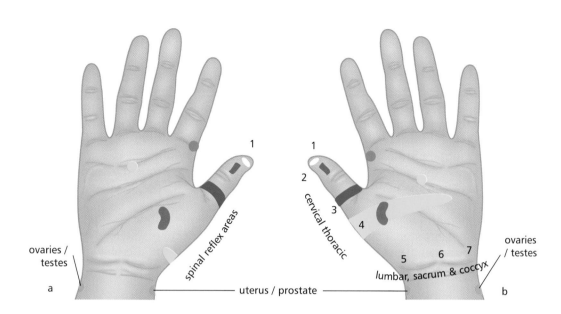

Figure 5/3: Areas on the hands corresponding to the main chakras and associated endocrine glands, plantar view; a. right hand, b. left hand. (See Table 6).

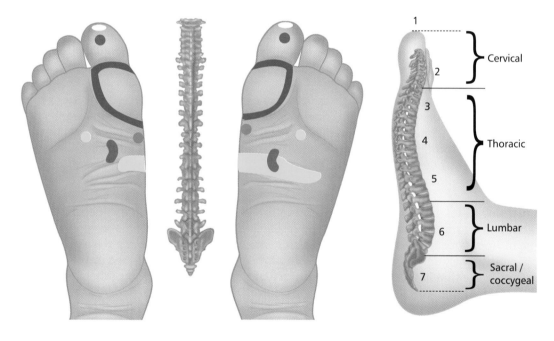

Figure 5/4: Areas on the feet corresponding to the main chakras and associated endocrine glands on the spine reflex area. (See Table 6).

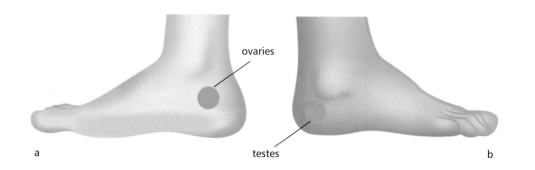

Figure 5/5: Location of the sixth chakra (gonads) on the foot; a) medial, b) lateral.

The abundance of body nerves is paralleled by the *nadis* network of fluid-like energies. Nadis are believed to be formed by fine threads of subtle energy matter. In that respect, they differ from the physical counterpart of the system of meridians.

Many thousands of these etheric channels of energy are believed to exist in the human body. They are interwoven with the physical nervous system. This interconnection with the nerves leads to the nadis affecting the type and quality of nerve impulses within the network of the brain, spinal cord and the peripheral nerves.

In summary, for optimum health, there needs to be an etheric / physical balance between the major chakras, the nadis network, the hormonal secretions from the glands of the endocrine system, and the nerve plexuses.

The chakras transform this energy of higher vibration into a lower vibrational physiological form that provides hormonal signals to the glands of the endocrine system. These glands then release minute quantities of their hormone into the bloodstream, thereby affecting the function of the whole physical body and emotions.

All organs of the body have their own energy frequency and those of similar frequency appear to be clustered, as with the solar plexus chakra and its association with and effect upon the stomach, liver, pancreas and gallbladder; all major players in the game of digestion. 'Food' for thought; to what extent might the solar plexus chakra have on the ability of the pancreas to produce insulin? The answer might give a clue to the increasing incidence of diabetes; particularly late onset diabetes. Could energy depletion of the chakra affect the body sufficiently to increase the risk? Could be worth investigation.

Chakras are not simply energy vortexes; they are centres of psychic perception. For example, the *brow* chakra, or *Ajna* chakra, is known as 'the third eye' in Eastern culture, signifying its relationship with intuition and foresight. Also, they transform and convey energy, in a stepped-down form, from the spiritual, mental and astral levels. For good health there needs to be sufficient energy flow in the meridians and that they remain balanced, one with another, throughout the system.

A machine exists that is capable of measuring this energy flow through the meridians. It was developed by the Japanese subtle energy researcher Hiroshi Motoyama and glorified in the title of *Apparatus for Meridian Identification*[4] which, fortunately, became the acronym AMI. It is an extremely sensitive machine capable of measuring the flow of ions in the interstitial layer of tissue that lies just beneath the surface of the skin. By this means it became possible to show that the patterns of flowing ions corresponded with the paths of acupuncture meridians, that have been known for thousands of years in Eastern countries.

Motoyama's findings, via the output of the AMI were confirmed by specialists using pulse diagnosis, one of the traditional diagnostic methods of oriental medicine. These findings are recorded at the California Institute for Human Science, Encinitas, California, which was the American centre for Motoyama's research.

Their existence is supported also by the work of Dr. Valerie Hunt[5], who originally set out to study the therapeutic energy effects of Rolfing. She used more conventional measuring equipment normally associated with measuring the electrical potential of muscles. Bio-electrical changes in areas of the skin that corresponded to the chakras was measured and recorded. She found high frequency electrical oscillations at these points that had not been recorded previously. For example, the normal frequency of brain waves is between 0 and 100 cps (cycles per second); muscle frequency is up to approximately 225 cps and heart frequency can reach 250 cps. The readings Dr. Hunt observed and recorded from the respective positions of the chakras were from 100 to 1600 – much higher than had been found previously to radiate from the body.

Just as intriguing was the contribution of Rosalyn Bruyere to the study by Dr. Hunt. Rosalyn Bruyere was a trained psychic observer and clairvoyant who could observe changes of aura. So Bruyere observed the subject's subtle energy field whilst the chakras were monitored electronically – using the EMG (electromyography) electrodes. During these observations she was denied knowledge of the electronic readings coming from the electrodes attached to the skin at the various chakra points, so that her observation remained unbiased.

The outcome was that Bruyere observed that colour changes coincided with the electrode readings. Over a sufficiently significant period of time it was found that each colour of the aura was associated with a different wave pattern recorded at the chakra points on the skin of the participants.

In practice, the valuable thing is that intricate and subtle systems – such as meridians of energy flow and chakra nadi networks – evidently exist which link the etheric body with the physical body. We need to be aware of them and for them to form part of our thinking when we take a holistic approach to a patient's whole wellbeing and quality of life.

Relating these thoughts to the therapy of reflexology serves to enhance what many practitioners have found (without seeking it), that if we take our hands a small distance from the feet or hands, a warmth or 'glow' can be felt by the patient. Since heat is a form of energy, it demonstrates the existence of an energy field that surrounds the feet and hands and, indeed, the whole body. This phenomenon can now be placed in this broader context.

Up until this point we have considered a physical-etheric interface and, to some extent, the associated physiological aspects; in a sense we have looked from the etheric to the body (inwards). There is, however, a further outer shroud beyond the etheric layer and energy transfer occurs between these outer levels. In addition, the level of subtleness seems to increase as we move 'outwards' from the physical body.

At this stage, scientists usually get worried and are definitely sceptical about this whole concept. I suspect this is because, as yet, we have not got the advanced equipment to measure its existence – they cannot get hold of it and prove its existence to their satisfaction. It's one of life's oldest human reactions to ridicule and dismiss that which we do not yet understand, often accompanied by fear of the unknown or by fear of the financial consequences upon established organisations with a vested interest in the outcome.

Therefore, we are now in the 'grey area' in the opinion of many Western scientists and we are in the 'partial vacuum' that seems to exist between Western and Far Eastern belief systems – particularly regarding the maintenance of good health and vitality. Historically, the lack of acceptance of the interrelationship between the physical body and physiological and endocrine balance of the body is due, in part, to the separation of the various religions and science thousands of years ago. The astral body or shroud of subtle energy is about emotion and instinct; the feeling of 'I've been here before' comes into this category. We are talking here of spirit rather than physical being.

At the spiritual level, desires come from the soul (our core-self that survives beyond death of the physical form that we 'rent' whilst on this planet earth). These desires are believed to enter the etheric body through the heart chakra[1]. Where there is no link with the soul, the energy passes to the solar plexus and is expressed as the desires of the personality.

There appears to be a reflective aspect of the astral body in as much as, if we wake in a positive frame of mind; feeling good, the whole day seems to go well and we meet and work with people of similar cheerful, positive, disposition. Conversely, the opposite can be true when there are days, months even, when whatever we do, nothing seems to go right.

Heart's Energy

It is now known that our heart creates the body's strongest electromagnetic field and this accounts, for example, for the perceptible difference in appearance of a corpse as distinct from a body asleep. The corpse has no electromagnetic energy because of the ceased heart beat; a physical manifestation of no energy.

Dr. William Collinge, in his book *Subtle Energy*[6] also claims that the heart's electromagnetic field expands and strengthens when we experience love, compassion and caring. It is interesting that the latter two aspects form important parts of good health care and that they have a direct influence upon our electromagnetic energy.

This triggers the thought that, maybe, ME sufferers would benefit from a loving, caring and compassionate relationship and environment. But then again, I guess we all would!

Each heartbeat produces a wave of electromagnetic energy that pulses outwards in all directions; like the ripples in a pond when we lob a stone into it. In a loving relationship, one of the benefits of 'opening our heart' is that this expression of our innermost feelings causes the waves to become more coherent. Normally, there is some irregularity in the wave pattern, but feelings of love results in these waves becoming more uniform and consistent[7].

Research at the Institute of Heartmath in Boulder Creek, California, found that this greater coherence and regularity reflects similar greater balance and harmony in our nervous system[8] and is associated with improved immunity[7]. This greater regularity is similar to the re-balancing and constitutional harmonisation towards homeostasis produced by reflexology treatments.

Dr. Rollin McCraty of the Institute of Heartmath found that our heart is capable of producing approximately 2.5 watts of electromagnetic power with each beat; enough to power a small radio transmitter. The heart's magnetic field is about a thousand times stronger than that of the brain. He claims that electrocardial energy can be found in every cell of our body, from our toes to our ears.

The work of McCraty and his colleagues revealed that an electrocardiogram will record changed waveforms of the heart caused by changes in our thoughts and emotions[7]; stress, depression, anxiety or frustration causes the wave pattern to become more irregular and incoherent.

Conversely, when we are calm and at peace with the world, the heart's energy waveform is smoother and more coherent. A fascinating by-product is that other oscillators – chakras – tend to come into balance, promoting optimal health and wellbeing.

It is hardly surprising, therefore, that the heart energy pulse reaches out beyond the skin and radiates in our surrounding space. A magnetometer can measure this electromagnetic field up to five feet away from the body and this explains, perhaps, what spiritual healers can 'feel' as they work around and at a distance from the body. It also suggests that we can actually detect 'vibes' radiating from those around us and why those who are fearful, angry, etc. can drain our energy. Equally, those who are positive and full of joy and optimism have an uplifting effect.

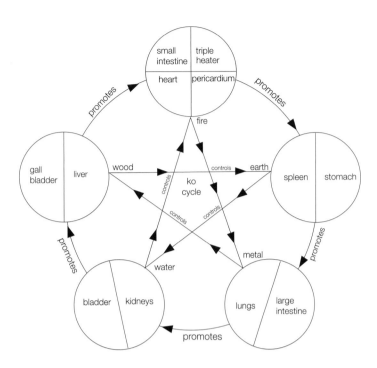

Figure 5/6: The law of the five elements.

From the Traditional Chinese Medicine (TCM) viewpoint there are many aspects of this form of re-balancing energy, or healing. Four aspects of this re-balancing of interest to the reflexologist are the Law of the Five Elements, Acupressure Points, Yin and Yang (pronounced 'inn' and 'arng'), and the Time Clock.

Law of the Five Elements

The energy of the universe, as regarded by Ayurvedic medicine and by TCM, is made up of five major Elements. Their interrelationship explains life's processes and influences upon our bodily functions and health, in relation to nature. This reference to nature is emphasised by each Element being named after some of the basic components of the natural world.

In Ayurvedic medicine the Elements are called Earth, Water, Fire, Air and Ether; in TCM these same Elements are called Water, Fire, Wood, Metal and Earth (the Cosmological Cycle). It is a matter of personal choice as to which nomenclature we use. To me, the Chinese names seem the most fundamental and because reflexology is believed to have originated from China and the Far East, it is the system that will be used here.

For a balanced personality and for balanced total wellbeing, all five Elements need to be in balance, thus providing unobstructed, healthy energy-flow in a kind of network or mesh as represented diagrammatically (see Figure 5/6). Each organ is regarded as being in one of the five Elements; the Yang organs on the outside and the Yin organs on the inside, with the Yin / Yang couple opposite each other. The 'Ko' Cycle is said to be the Control Cycle, with the 'Shen' Cycle as the Creation Cycle. The five Elements are not chemical elements but rather aspects of life, nature and constitution.

Referring to Figure 5/6, the Creation, or 'Shen' Cycle shows that Fire produces Earth (by burning wood, the ash is returned to the earth); Earth produces Metal (metallic ore comes from the earth); Metal produces Water (springs of water are found by mineral deposits); Water produces Wood (trees grow by absorbing water through their roots) and so on around the Cycle.

With the Control, or 'Ko' Cycle, each Element has a controlling influence upon the succeeding Element; acting as checks and balances. If an Element is too weak, it can absorb energy from another. Figure 5/6 shows it as a Control Cycle whereby Wood controls Earth (the roots of trees bind soil together, and prevents its erosion); Earth controls Water (dams, depth of rivers and streams); Water controls Fire (water can extinguish fire); Fire controls Metal (fire can melt metal) and Metal controls Wood (axes, drills, planing machines remove wood). The Cycle is continuous and in conjunction with the Creation Cycle. The significance of these two Cycles is that they form the basis of the application of acupuncture treatment.

Again referring to Figure 5/6, the Creation Cycle shows that the heart, small intestine and triple heater support the spleen and stomach; they, in turn, support the lungs and large intestine and so on around to the gallbladder and liver supporting the heart, small intestine and triple heater. It is a Cycle of interdependence, one (or two) organs with another.

Probably, the acupuncturist is more likely to be presented with having to address a degree of illness or imbalance, with accompanying signs and symptoms. The focus would then be upon the Control Cycle – but not exclusively, because of the interdependencies. For example, if the energy of the heart is low, it can affect the lungs and large intestine; low bladder and kidney energy can affect the heart. We see similarities in Western conventional medical practice. If there is low cardial output, it leads to lung congestion via pulmonary congestion, which can lead to reduced liver function.

Figure 5/6, therefore, serves as a very brief and basic illustration of a small part of the philosophy of acupuncture and acupressure and because reflexologists use pressure on specific points it is useful if not vital, that we have some knowledge – a working knowledge – of this philosophy.

Acupressure Points

Meridians as channels of subtle energy are connected with the therapies of acupuncture (needles) and acupressure (no needles). Each of these therapies treat specific points on the body's surface to release or rebalance the flow of energy along defined channels within human anatomy. These specific points are called *acupoints* or *tsubos*; the meridian lines 'join' these various points forming a network of energy channels.

There are 14 named meridians of which 11 are associated with organs identified in mainstream medicine and 2 that are not[9] (the third meridian, the triple heater, is the 'linking factor' connecting the organ functions). In addition, there are a further 6 meridians that are composites of the others, making a grand total of 20 meridians. We are fortunate in reflexology to restrict ourselves only to the points that are identified on the foot and lower limb (below the knee) and to the hand and forearm (to the elbow). It is not the intention to make reflexologists into pseudo acupuncturists so we will confine ourselves to working on the feet and hands.

The Chinese have practiced acupressure on themselves and disseminated with other cultures for over 5000 years, as a way of maintaining health and vitality. Their philosophy is that defined channels of life force energy (Qi) exist and that application of pressure, at specific points, frees or clears this energy-flow. Conversely, if these points hold blockages it has an adverse effect upon our general health. Qi is said to exist in every cell of the body and that its cumulative influence is as an all-pervading energy. Its flow can be manipulated to greatest effect at the specific acu-points; in particular those between knee and toes (lower limb) and between elbow and fingers (lower arm). These are 'command' points and there are one or two 'great' points that exist in each meridian (energy channel). These 'great' points are used more frequently than others because the experience of acupuncturists and acupressure therapists suggest that they are more effective than other points.

Yin and Yang

The Yin-Yang theory is an ancient Chinese conceptual framework that serves as a means for viewing and understanding the world. It is the foundation for understanding all phenomena and, in the context of Chinese medicine, for understanding health and disease. Yin is the cloudy or shady side of the hill, and Yang the sunny side. On the Yang side it is light, warm and people are working, while on the shady side it is cold, dark and everyone is resting. The interaction of Yin and Yang gives rise to Qi, which is the invisible life energy that flows through the meridians around the body (*see* page 106). The even circulation of Qi around the body is essential for health.

However, Yin and Yang are relative terms. Something is Yin (or Yang) only in relation to something else. It doesn't make sense to talk of Yin except in relation to Yang; they are opposing but also complementary. The two make up the full picture, without the one the other is incomplete.

There are five main ways in which Yin and Yang are related to one another. They: i. oppose one another; ii. complement one another; iii. can consume one another; iv. can transform into one another; v. can be further divided into Yin and Yang. In addition, they are infinitely divisible.

In the body, disease is caused by an imbalance of Yin and Yang. Therefore, disease can be treated by correcting this imbalance and allowing the body to heal itself. As reflexologists, we are used to the concept that, as with most therapies, the acute needs to be addressed before the chronic aspects can be detected and treated; the 'peeling the onion' concept.

Traditional Chinese Medicine (TCM) Time Clock

The flow of Qi energy within and along the meridians varies throughout the 24 hour cycle whilst adhering to a definite and repetitive pattern. Hence, in theory, there are specific periods when certain organs and body systems are at peak energy or at a low energy. These periods are of approximately 2 hours duration in each 24 hours. For example, heart energy peaks at 12 noon and is at the least at 24 hours (midnight). This knowledge is useful in knowing the hour of the day when treatment would have its greatest benefit. But getting patients to attend during the night has a large element of unreality. Like so many things, common sense and suitable compromise has to be used to apply the knowledge during normal working hours. Equally, it is useful to know that it may be normal for a particular organ or system to display certain symptoms at specific times of the day and not others. In short, it is another tool in the reflexologist's toolbag of knowledge and experience that can be utilised with patients whose condition is proving difficult to overcome or which appears to defy logical deduction.

To avoid getting too far from reflexology, this is as far as we take it. The important thing is that we are aware of the existence of these subtle energies and influences and their place in the overall picture of health as seen by our present knowledge, study and experience.

No comment about body energy would be complete without mentioning the most advanced and comprehensive therapy I have experienced; electronic vibrational medicine. It uses the Harmonic Translation System (HTS), as pioneered and developed by Dr. Peter Moscow in the USA. He is President of the US Psychotronics Association and of the Electronic Medicine Association whose work in the UK is co-ordinated by Mr. John Morley-Kirk who is also an extremely competent reflexologist. John served for a number of years as Director of the Midlands Region of the UK division of the International Institute of Reflexology. We mentioned earlier that the body possesses its own, individual vibrations. The Harmonic Translation System utilises this fact. Everything on our planet has its own vibration, whether it is a flower, vitamin, enzyme, herb or homoeopathic tincture.

HTS can analyse every part of the body in great detail, taking an individual's overall vitality energy level as an overall benchmark. It will reveal the bioenergy level (vitality) of every organ, gland and body part, together with the level of stress that part is suffering.

Having identified where a problem (or problems) exist, it provides the process of restoring healthy bioenergy balance by selecting from a vast bank of herbs, homoeopathic tinctures, flower essences, metals, crystals and sound pulses, to build a programme of sound and visual patterns onto a video-tape that the patient uses for the prescribed number of days and at the prescribed best times of day.

For those who may be intrigued by this glimpse into the world of subtle energy and vibrational medicine, and would like a more detailed explanation and discussion, I suggest you refer to the references at the end of this chapter.

On page 120 is a *Confidential Patient Record* which I found very useful and practical because you can chat to your patient whilst ticking boxes to build a simple profile of your patient's emotional state. It's important to take the ticked boxes as a whole and to avoid judging the patient in any way whatsoever. From a practical point of view, it saves time writing and allows eye contact to be maintained throughout discussion. You can then study it and make any additional notes post visit. If you would like to try this, please feel free to save yourself time by copying the tabulation.

For those who wish to expand their knowledge of the aspects of energy discussed in this chapter, I recommend the postgraduate seminars of Lillian Tibshraeny-Morten '*12 Meridians and the 5 Elements*' (*see* Useful Addresses), the seminars of Energy Works (Anna Jeoffroy and Philip Salmon) and John Cross's well-illustrated and comprehensive book '*Acupressure*' [9] and the work done under the auspices of the Electronic Medicine Association (*see* Useful Addresses).

		ASSOCIATED					
Chakra	Location	Endocrine Gland (Hormone)	Nerve Plexus	Sense	Quality	Colour	Sanskrit
1. Crown	Top of head	Pineal (melatonin)	Cerebral cortex	Spirit	Spirituality / liberation	Violet, gold or white	7. Sahasrara
2. Third eye	Slightly above & between eyebrows	Pituitary (stimulating hormones)	Hypothalamus / pituitary	Thought	Vision, thought & reason	Indigo	6. Ajna
3. Throat	Throat (C3–C5)	Thyroid (thyroxine)	Cervical ganlia	Sound	Communication	Blue	5. Visuddha
4. Heart	Centre of thoracic cavity, behind the heart	Thymus (thymosin)	Cardiac plexus	Touch	Love / compassion	Green	4. Anahata
5. Solar plexus	Base of sternum	Pancreas (insulin)	Solar plexus	Sight	Power / control	Yellow	3. Manipuraka
6. Sacral	Lower abdomen / sacrum	Ovaries / testes (oestrogen / progesterone / testosterone)	Sacral	Taste	Centering sexual urge (libido)	Orange	2. Svadhisthana
7. Base	Perineum (men) – between genitals / anus; cervix (women) – between vagina / uterus	Adrenals (corticosteroids / adrenaline)	Sacro-coccygeal	Smell	Will to survive / grounding	Red	1. Muladhara

Table 7. Summary of Chakras and the Links to our Glands, Senses and Life Quality. NOTE: The number of the Chakras in the first column refer to the Western system and those on the far right (Sanskrit) refer to the Eastern system.

Do Not Forget

The main areas of the spine – the backbone of health – associated with the endocrine system are: **C1** Pituitary; **C7** Thyroid; **T7** Pancreas (dual role with digestion); **T9** Adrenals; **L3** Gonads.

It is a kind of telephone number: 17793, and can be used in association with the meridian points of the following section.

The Main Meridians and Acupressure Points

The purpose of the following pages is to provide a summary of the meridian points relevant to reflexology and, also, to provide a working reference. There are great points for each meridian that have greater energetic influence than the other respective points, and they can have more than one function. For easy reference, asterisks (*) identify these points.

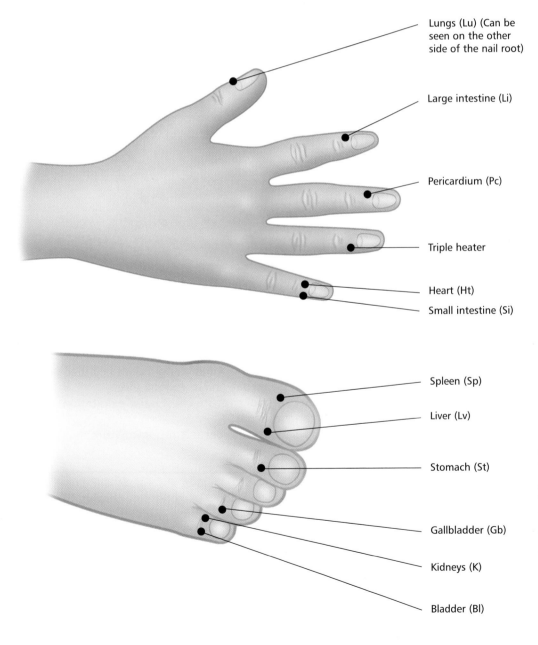

Lungs (Lu) (Can be seen on the other side of the nail root)

Large intestine (Li)

Pericardium (Pc)

Triple heater

Heart (Ht)

Small intestine (Si)

Spleen (Sp)

Liver (Lv)

Stomach (St)

Gallbladder (Gb)

Kidneys (K)

Bladder (Bl)

Figure 5/7: Some very useful meridian points which are at the extremity of their respective meridians. Reproduced with the kind permission of Mr. Anthony Porter, Director ART Training.

Heart, Lung and Pericardium Main Meridian Notes

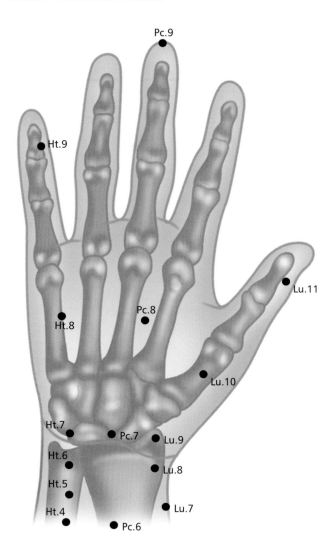

Figure 5/7: Main heart, lung and pericardium meridian points (palmar view).

Ht.7*   A great point for the release of emotional 'blockage'; a consequent 'release' point; reduces irritability; calms; helps overcome insomnia and reduces cardiac pain.

Ht.8   Clears palpitations, tachycardia, sore throat, thirst, tongue ulcers.

Ht.9   Emergency point for heart attack or stroke; acute chest pain; palpitations; circulation generally. Revives consciousness.

Lu.7   Oxygen point. Emotional grief / sadness and chronic respiratory problems.

Lu.8   Throat problems.

Lu.9   Throat coughs and voice.

Lu.10   Cough, asthma, sore throat.

Lu.11   Resuscitates consciousness and most commonly used for sore throats.

Pc.6*   Insomnia (together with heart point Ht.7); palpitation (with Ht.9); chest pain; nausea – particularly in early pregnancy and also for travel sickness.

Pc.7   Palpitations (with Ht.9); insomnia (with Ht.7); cardiac pain (with Ht.9); stomach ache.

Pc.8   Halitosis; gastritis.

Pc.9   Stroke / cardiac pain (with Ht.9); palpitations (with Ht.9 and Pc.7); heart burn.

Stomach Main Meridian Notes

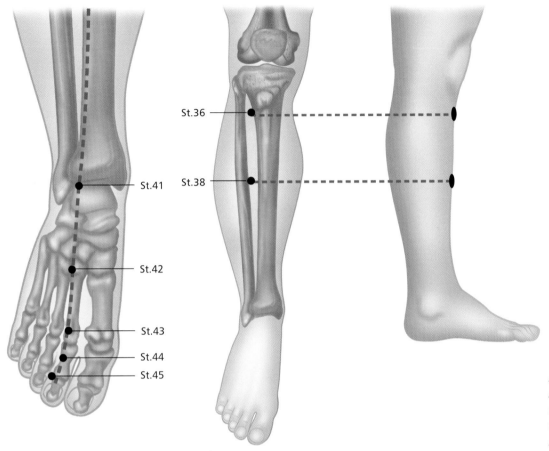

a   b

Figure 5/8: (a) Stomach main meridian points; (b) two great points on the main stomach meridian.

St.36* (Located one patient's finger width lateral to the anterior crest of the tibial bone; between it and the fibula – "in the valley between the bones"). Affects upper gastro-intestinal conditions, i.e. nausea, vomiting. Note: heavy stimulation of this point can produce vomit of stomach contents. Conversely, gentle pressure has a calming effect upon stomach pain (gastralgia). This particular point influences numerous signs and symptoms generally. If there was only time to work one point, this would be it.

St.38 Can help overcome pain and stiffness of the shoulder.

St.41 Ankle joint conditions; leg paralysis / cramps; abdominal disorders; thirst; dizziness; vertigo, and headache.

St.42 Used to treat weaknesses in the stomach and spleen with symptoms such as poor appetite, digestion, and tiredness.

St.43 Regulates the stomach function and helps in the dispersal of any oedema in the body generally.

St.44 Throat soreness / discomfort*; headache; toothache. Also treats symptoms such as burning epigastric pain, and halitosis.

St.45 Used in cases of mental restlessness, agitation, and insomnia.

* Important that patient sees their doctor for clinical check / diagnosis.

Spleen Main Meridian Notes

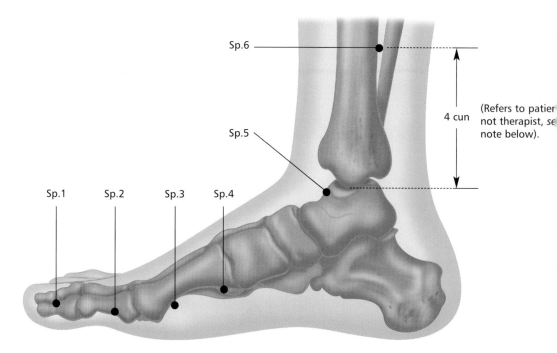

Figure 5/9: Spleen main meridian points (medial view).

Spleen energy is responsible for peristalsis.

Sp.1   Calms the mind and regulates blood flow. Useful in treating excessive uterine bleeding, haemorrhoids.

Sp.2   Gastric pain; diarrhoea; constipation, i.e. regulates bowel function.

Sp.3   Lack of appetite; difficulty urinating; vaginal discharge. Tiredness, obesity, abdominal distension, and loose stools. Also used for poor concentration and sleepiness.

Sp.4   Tones the meridian generally. Relates the flow of Ki and blood. Chronic pain, nausea, sickness, and menstruation. Also infertility.

Sp.5   Mainly used for foot, leg, knee and ankle problems, but also abdominal distension, and constipation.

Sp.6*   **Do not use if the patient is known to be pregnant.** Strengthens spleen energy; assists liver function; assists detoxification of kidneys; regulates menses (menstrual flow); alleviates pain; assists lymphatic function. Used for tiredness, abdominal distension and pain, impotence, night sweats and restlessness.

A 'cun' was the measurement used in ancient China, long before imperial measure. It took account of individuality of patients, because the measurement is of the patient's thumb width or base of first and second finger width as shown below:

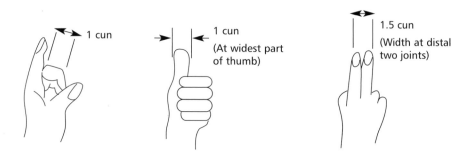

Large Intestine (Colon) Main Meridian Notes

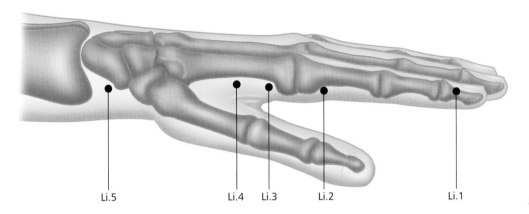

Li.5   Li.4   Li.3   Li.2   Li.1

Figure 5/10: Large intestine (colon) main meridian points.

Li.1   Numbness in fingers; toothache. Mainly used to treat acute pain, swelling and inflammation of the throat.

Li.2   Conjunctivitis, blurred vision; epistaxis (nosebleed).

Li.3   Pain relief.

Li.4*   This is the most important of the large intestine points and is contra indicated for pregnancy and menstruation, as it promotes labour and birth. Used for pain relief for face, head, shoulders and elbows; coughs; migraine; constipation, stomach troubles generally; toothache and lower jaw pain relief; pain relief of the back of the neck (dorsum) and occiput (the boney bumps at the back and base of the head); skin conditions – especially acne.

Li.5   Important point for problems of the wrist and thumb. Sited in the centre of the large depression between the tendons of extensor pollicis longus and brevis.

Note: Known as the 'analgesic point', it is a very influential point and has wide versatility. It can be used in association with other points, such as:

• With Lv.3 – acute pain / stress / headache / nervous tension.
• With Lu.7 – clears throat and chest congestion and pain.
• With Si.2 and Si.3 – control of nosebleeds.
• With Ht.7 – insomnia; nightmares.

Small Intestine Main Meridian Notes

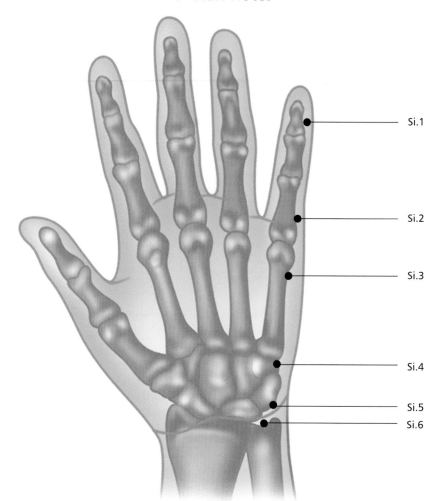

Figure 5/11: Small intestine main meridian points.

Si.1   Headache; pain in neck; active tonsillitis. Calms the mind, restores consciousness.

Si.2   Tinnitus ('ringing' or buzzing sensation in the ears); headache; numbness of the fingers (be suspicious – this can be caused by displacement or rotation of a cervical bone in the neck. If suspected **refer** to patient's doctor, osteopath or chiropractor).

Si.3*   Posterior shoulder pain; trigeminal neuralgia; elbow pain; metacarpal pain; headache; peripheral neuropathy of arm / hand. **This is a key point, in association with Bl.62 for the treatment of numerous spinal conditions.**

Si.4   Neck – rigidity; headache; wrist pain.

Si.5   Wrist pain; swelling of neck (check for swollen lymphatic glands by gentle touch).

Si.6   Blurred vision; shoulder pain; pain in elbow and / or arm. Stops pain anywhere along the small intestine channel.

Note: Si points can address the inability to rotate the head the full 180° left to right and vice versa. Can help alleviate pain in testes that can be connected to back condition (wise to **refer**, in case the pain has a sinister cause).

Kidney Main Meridian Notes

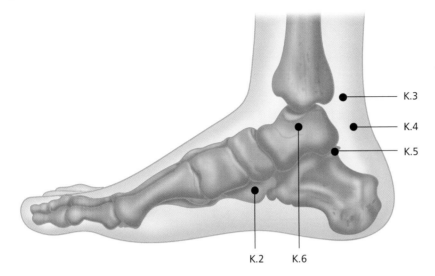

a

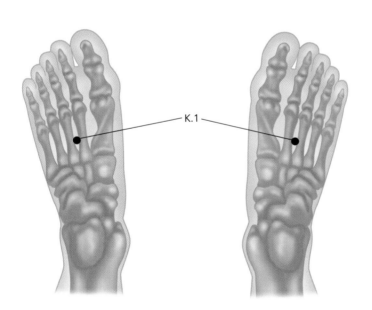

b

Figure 5/12: Kidney main meridian points; (a) medial view; (b) plantar view.

K.1   Mental disorders; severe anxiety; headache; dizziness; hypertension.

K.2   Irregular menstruation; prolapsed uterus.

K.3   Irregular menstruation; impotence; frequent urination (can be age-related), vertigo; tinnitus; pain in lower back; exhaustion; diminished hearing and sight.

K.4   Asthma; pain in lower back.

K.5   Irregular menses; prolapsed uterus.

K.6*   Night sweats; sore throat; insomnia; hot flushes; menopausal syndromes. It is a significant 'energy point'; consequently, it should be palpated for chronic fatigue syndrome or when major tiredness is a patient's concern or symptom.

Note: The major emotion of kidney is fear – including the reluctance to 'let go'.

Kidney dysfunction can be caused by physical and / or mental overwork; old age; chronic illness; severe acute illness; excessive sexual activity in males and multiple births in females.

Bladder Main Meridian Notes

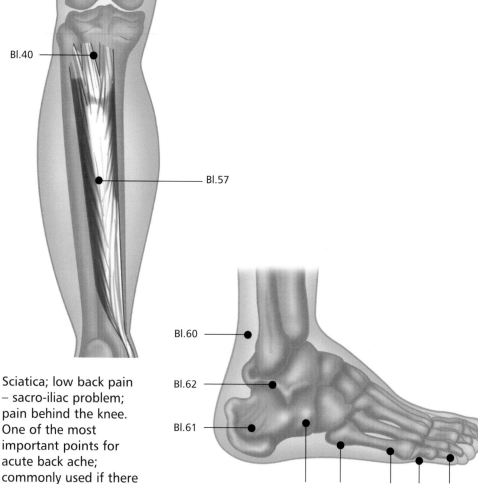

Figure 5/13: Bladder main meridian points.

Bl.40   Sciatica; low back pain – sacro-iliac problem; pain behind the knee.

Bl.57   One of the most important points for acute back ache; commonly used if there is pain, cramps or weakness of the calf and leg; sciatica or lumbar pain. Also treats haemorrhoids and dysmenorrhoea.

Bl.60   Chronic backache; headache; pains in neck and shoulders; menstrual problems.

Bl.61   Muscular atrophy of lower limbs; heel pain.

Bl.62*   Alleviates pain in low back (lumbar, sacrum); it is a major point for pain relief generally – including painful knee conditions; tendon problems and ankle disorders.

Bl.63   Relaxes muscles and tendons; backache; motor impairment of lower extremities.

Bl.64   Headache; rigidity of the neck.

Bl.65   Headache at nape of neck; stiff neck; blurred vision; backache.

Bl.66   Headaches and stiff necks.

Bl.67   Invigorates the mind; clears vision and, generally, 'refreshes the head'. Powerful effect on the uterus and is therefore contraindicated during pregnancy.

Note: For headaches generally:
If sited at forehead – stomach reflex area, plus St.41.
If temporal (either side of head) – gallbladder reflex area, plus Gb.41.
If at top of head – liver reflex area, plus Lv.2 and Lv.3.

Liver Main Meridian Notes

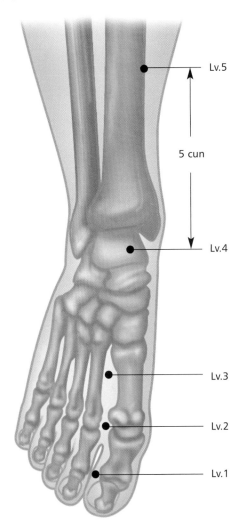

Lv.5

5 cun

Lv.4

Lv.3

Lv.2

Lv.1

Figure 5/14: Liver main meridian points.

Lv.1   Used to subdue internal wind and restore consciousness.

Lv.2   Headache; disturbed sleep; irritability.

Lv.3*   Excellent point for cramp (irrespective of location on body) particularly good for cramp of the calf muscle. Gentle touch only is needed, with no palpation or excitation. Calms nerves, eases headaches behind the eyes and hangovers; muscular tiredness; dizziness; insomnia; infertility; irregular menses. In summary, a very influential point.

Lv.4   Painful menses; vaginal discharge; urine retention. Effectively treats pain, swelling, and stiffness of the ankle.

Lv.5   Can help towards recovery from a stroke (in combination with other 'points' of bladder, kidneys and spleen). Important point for problems of the genitourinary organs.

Gallbladder Main Meridian Notes

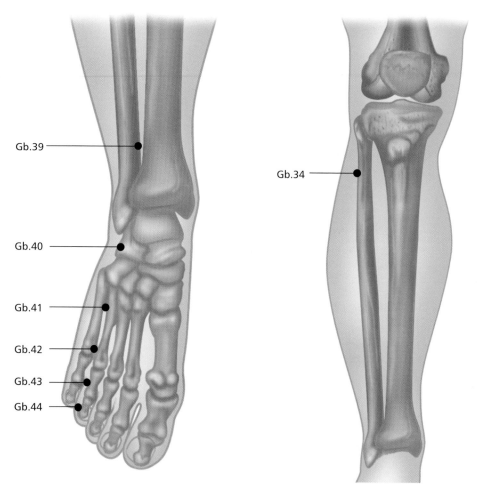

*Figure 5/15:
Gallbladder main
meridian points.*

Gb.34   Situated in the depression in front of (anterior) and below (inferior) to the head of the fibula – the smaller, lateral, shin bone. A very important point in the treatment of musculo-skeletal problems anywhere in the body. If this point is tender it indicates a tendon problem and, as such, is a good diagnostic tool alongside mainstream diagnostic techniques. Also abdominal pain, PMS, irritability, and sciatica.

Gb.39   Viewed from behind the fibula. Blood marrow disorders (e.g. chronic lymphatic leukaemia); pain in leg and / or ankle; neck pain and torticollis (twisted head / neck condition or wry neck which is the contraction of the sternocleidomastoid muscle – the neck muscle that has its origin at the sternum (breastbone) and clavicle (collarbone) and inserts at the mastoid process of the temporal – the bony bump you can feel behind and above the ear.

Gb.40   Arthritis and disorders of the ankle; neck pain.

Gb.41*   Mastitis; dysmenorrhoea (painful menstruation – often on first day of bleeding); lactation problems; pain in the feet.

Gb.42   Breast pain; pain and / or swelling of dorsum (top) of foot.

Gb.43   Headache and migraine, tinnitus, deafness and vertigo.

Gb.44   Stroke; deafness and tinnitus; vertigo; disorders of the eye (**always refer**); improves hearing and sight and calms the mind.

Note: Low gallbladder energy contributes to indecisiveness.

References

1. Gerber, R.: 1996. *Vibrational Medicine – New Choices for Healing Ourselves*. Bear & Co. (ISBN: 1 879181 28 2).
2. Pert, C. B.: 1997. *Molecules of Emotion*. Scribner. (ISBN: 0 684 8318 7 2).
3. Scott-Mumby, K.: 1999. *Virtual Medicine*. Thorsons, London. (ISBN: 0 7225 3823 5).
4. Jackson, A.: 1992. E*nergetic Medicine: A New Science of Healing*; Interview with Dr. Hiroshi Motoyama. *Share International Magazine,* 11(7): 5–7.
5. *Electronic Evidence of Auras, Chakras in UCLA Study. Brain / Mind Bulletin*, 3 (9) (March 1978).
6. William Collinge, W.: 1998. *Subtle Energy (Understanding the Life-Force Energies that Surround Us)*. Thorsons, London. (ISBN: 0 7225 3668 2).
7. Rein, G., Atkinson, M. and McCraty, R. In press: *The physiological and psychological effects of compassion and anger. Journal of Advancement in Medicine*.
8. McCraty, R., Atkinson, M. and Tiller, A.: 1994. *New electrophysiological correlates associated with intentional heart focus*. Unpublished manuscript, Institute of Heartmath, 14700 West Park Ave., Boulder Creek, CA 95006.
9. Cross, J. R.: 2000. *Acupressure – Clinical Applications in Musculo-skeletal Conditions*. Butterworth-Heinemann, London. (ISBN: 0 7506 4054 5).

Bibliography

Page, C.: 1992. *Frontiers of Health – Healing to Wholeness*. Daniel, UK. (ISBN: 0 8527 256 2).
Arewa, C. S.: 1998. *Opening to Spirit*. Thorsons, UK. (ISBN: 0 7225 3726 3).

Confidential Patient Record

Patient's Name: .... Sex: .... D.O.B.: ....

SYMPTOM		ELEMENT/S	ORGAN/S		EMOTION/S
Abdominal pain		Metal	Li		Anguish
Aching body		Earth	Sp		Obsessions
Anger		Wood	Li		Aggression / Depression
Angina		Fire	Pc		Joy
Ankle and lower leg pain		Wood	Gb		Aggression / Depression
Appetite, poor		Earth	Sp		Obsessions
Arm pain, medial		Metal	Lu		Anguish
Asthma		Fire / Water	K; Pc		Fear / Obsessions
Axilla pain		Fire	Peri		Joy
Back pain, ref. testicles		Fire	Si		Joy
Bed wetting		Water	Bl; K		Fear
Behaviour, irrational		Fire	Ht		Joy
Borborygmus		Fire	Si		Joy
Bowel movement, abnormal		Fire	Si		Joy
Breast pain		Wood	Li		Aggression / Depression
Cardiac pain		Fire	Pc		Joy
Cardiac palpitations		Fire	Pc		Joy
Clavicle pain		Metal	Lu		Anguish
Cold sores, mouth / upper lip		Fire	Si		Joy
Complexion, blue / purple		Fire	Ht		Joy
Complexion, pale		Fire	Ht		Joy
Concentration, difficult		Fire	Ht		Joy
Constipation		Metal / Earth	Li; St		Anguish / Obsessions
Cough		Water / Metal	K; Lu		Fear / Anguish
Cough, dry		Fire	Pc		Joy
Cystitis		Water	Bl		Fear
Deafness		Wood / Water / Heart	Gb; K; Si		Anger / Fear / Joy
Dental problems		Water	K		Fear
Digestive disturbance		Fire	St; Si		Joy
Dizziness		Water	K		Fear
Dreaming, excessive		Fire	Ht		Joy
Dysmenorrhoea, painful		Wood	Gb		Aggression / Depression
Dyspnea		Metal	Lu		Anguish
Ejaculation, premature		Water	K		Fear
Eye problems, dry		Wood	Li		Aggression / Depression
Eye problems, red		Wood	Li		Aggression / Depression
Face, red – congestion		Fire	Ht; Pc		Joy
Fatigue		Earth	Sp		Obsessions
Forgetfulness		Fire	Ht		Joy
Gas		Earth	St		Obsessions
Gums, swollen		Metal	Li		Anguish
Gynaecological problems		Wood	Li		Aggression / Depression
Haemorrhoids		Metal	Li		Anguish
Hair loss		Water	K		Fear
Halitosis		Metal	Li		Anguish
Head movement, restricted		Fire	Si		Joy
Headache		Earth / Water	St; Bl		Obsessions / Fear

SYMPTOM		ELEMENT/S	ORGAN/S		EMOTION/S
Headache, back of head		Water	Gb		Fear
Headache, temporal		Wood	Li		Aggression / Depression
Heartburn		Fire	Pc		Joy
Hysteria		Fire	Ht		Joy
Impotency		Water	K		Fear
Infertility		Water / Wood	K; Li		Fear / Aggression / Depression
Insomnia		Fire	Ht		Joy
Irritability		Wood	Li		Aggression / Depression
Jaundice		Wood	Li		Aggression / Depression
Knee pain		Earth	St		Joy
Lactation problems		Water	Gb		Fear
Lasitude		Earth	Sp		Obsessions
Laughter, uncontrollable		Fire	Pc		Joy
Leg and ankle pain		Wood	Gb		Aggression / Depression
Mastitis		Water	K		Fear
Memory, poor		Fire	Ht		Joy
Menstrual problems		Water	K		Fear
Migraine		Metal	Li		Anguish
Muscle pain		Earth	Sp		Obsessions
Nails, brittle		Wood	Li		Aggression / Depression
Neck rigidity		Water	Bl		Fear
Night emissions		Water	K		Fear
Nose bleeds		Water	Bl		Fear
Nose, runny / blocked		Metal	Li		Anguish
Oedema (lower leg)		Earth	Sp		Obsessions
Phlegm		Earth	Sp		Obsessions
PMS / PMT		Wood	Li		Aggression / Depression
Prostatitis		Water	Bl		Fear
Restlessness		Fire	Ht		Joy
Saliva, increased		Earth	St		Obsessions
Shoulder pain		Metal	Lu		Anguish
Shoulder pain, top / back		Metal	Li		Anguish
Skin problems		Metal	Lu		Anguish
Sperm count, low		Water	K		Fear
Stools, loose		Metal	Li		Anguish
Taste, bitter		Wood	Li		Aggression / Depression
Temperature problems		Fire	St; Si; Bl		Joy
Testicular pain		Fire	Si		Joy
Thinking, unclear		Fire	Ht		Joy
Throat, sore		Metal	Lu		Anguish
Throat, sore, chronic		Earth	St		Obsessions
Tinnitus		Wood / Water / Fire	Gb; K; SI		Anger / Fear / Joy
Tiredness		Earth	Sp		Obsessions
Toothache		Metal	Li		Anguish
Urination, frequent		Water	Bl		Fear
Urination, painful		Water	Bl		Fear
Urination, retention		Water	Bl		Fear
Vertigo		Wood / Water	Gb; K; Li		Aggression / Depression / Fear
Vision, blurred		Water / Wood	Bl; Gb		Fear / Aggression / Depression
Voice loss		Metal	Lu		Anguish
Wheezing		Metal	Lu		Anguish

Chapter 6

Research – Why and How?

This chapter is intended to give a brief introduction only to the topic of research which would merit a complete book by itself.

Why carry out research at all? I suggest it is to advance our knowledge and understanding and to present the outcome in a clear, concise form, capable of replication by others and thus produce the same or very similar outcome.

It seems that a great deal of research focuses upon verifying outcomes known already to many patients whose collective experience is anecdotal evidence and that this is regarded as insufficiently rigorous. I suspect this argument masks an underlying reason – that the collective and collated opinion and experience of numerous patients' benefits from treatment is not trusted. Certain factions within our society, therefore, set out to prove or disprove claims made to a level that satisfies themselves. Only then are they willing to lend their support to a particular therapy, procedure or treatment. In some instances this can be an expensive way of 're-inventing the wheel'. Surely the place of research is to find out the why and how, not the if; particularly when there are buckets full of anecdotal evidence that a therapy works. It is pointless spending money to prove what many know already. Not just know but have experienced for themselves – patients are not stupid; cynics are stupid when they fail to accept the evidence of their eyes and ears. What they imply is that they do not trust the opinion, experience and judgment of anyone else!

Eliminating bias is difficult. Eliminating financial vested interest in an outcome is difficult and can be masked behind a research-funding organisation. Eliminating distortion of method is also difficult, because we cannot avoid the individuality of personality and constitution. For example, it is well-known that someone of positive outlook determined to get well is more likely to respond to treatment than a thoroughly demoralised, negative person. For these reasons and others of human fallibility, it is a fallacy to talk of 'pure' research. Much that claims to be scientific is statistical analysis written up in the jargon of academia.

However, this should not deter us, my plea is that we accept these unavoidable variances; having set out to reduce them so that any outcome has minimal distortion. My argument is against only those who would have us believe that funded university research is, by title, somehow 'purer' than that undertaken outside of that setting.

So, let us consider some key issues in a constructive, open-minded, framework.

Practitioners of any health discipline are enthusiastic about their specialism and have, consequently, an in-built bias towards it. Therefore, when doing research it is difficult for us to stand aside from that bias; yet, if others are to be convinced of the validity of our findings, we must strive for unbiased consistency. Other pitfalls are error and confusion that can hinder research being rigorous and convincing.

The whole picture or climate of research can be confusing only because researchers have developed a language and procedures of their own. One can only suspect that this is a ploy to maintain exclusivity. To be fair, it might be the consequence of the 'newness' of their work. Lawyers, accountants, designers, information technology specialists all have their protective, specialist language. So we must make the effort to learn the language of research and the following introduces some of the words and terminology to be found amongst the undergrowth of the confusion trail.

Research has two broad approaches; *qualitative* research relies upon the written word and the accuracy of description. *Quantitative* research measures things and expresses them numerically in answer to specific questions.

Reflexology therapy raises many questions – particularly in clarifying the *protocol* – the basis for applications for financial support.

It is the working schedule of a research project and must be as clear and unambiguous as possible. The great deal of time, effort and cost in working out this stage brings proportional reward later in the total process.

Typical examples of the questions that are raised by a reflexology research project would include:

- How long would each treatment last?
- How many treatments are to be given to each patient?
- Which foot chart would be used as a reference throughout?
- Would treatment include the hands as well as the feet?
- What pressure is to be used?
- What type of reflexology, i.e. technique, is to be used?
- What are the boundaries of age of the patients?
- Are clinically diagnosed conditions to be used?
- If so, what conditions?
- How are we going to simulate a treatment for these in the control group?

This list is not exhaustive, and I am sure you can think of many more questions that would be relevant to a research project.

In considering some of the questions we have mentioned or hinted at, a few more words and phrases of the researchers' world occur.

One way of deciphering what exactly caused an improvement in a patient's condition is to use a control group in what is known as a *controlled trial.*

Case histories – the description of patients who improved following treatment – have their place. But, can we be sure that the improvement was due only to reflexology? Was the patient's diet unaltered, for example? Did the patient have morale boosting good news at about the same time? It is very hard to ensure that perfectly normal aspects of life do not distort recorded outcomes.

A second approach would be to have a group of patients with the same presenting symptoms and signs with whom we can compare outcomes from closely defined treatments. This forms a *cohort study*; it is one in which we treat a series of patients with the same condition and measure defined aspects of their condition before and then after treatment. This demands a way of measuring the condition accurately and with consistency sufficient to produce *reliability* and *validity*. Special *outcome measures* have been developed that have been demonstrated to be valid and reliable and we should use these proven techniques whenever possible.

Cohort studies also introduce the need for the researched population to be of sufficient size as to be statistically significant. That is, the patient's improvement is greater than would have been expected by chance variation.

The *controlled trial* helps to clarify what produced the benefit. The groups for comparison should be allocated without any bias by random selection. This then provides us with a *Randomised Controlled Trial (RCT)*. Probably it is the most accurate procedure in terms of establishing *evidence-based* efficacy of touch therapies used alongside mainstream medical practice.

The simplest form of RCT is when one group receives reflexology and the other does not. Any improvement recorded for the group receiving treatment must be because of the therapy. Or was it? What of the effect of receiving sympathetic attention? What of the effect of the empathy between therapist and patient; particularly the trust of the professionalism of the therapist by the patient? But these *non-specific effects* apply equally to allopathic health as they do to complementary health care; so let us not get too excited about that over which we can exercise little control.

This does, however, raise the aspect that reflexology – like most of the 'touch' therapies – has three components. The effect of treating the various points on the feet and hands correctly in relation to the specific reflexology treatment techniques being used throughout the study; the comfort of being touched; the relaxed state induced by the combination of the two.

A way of controlling the *non-specific effects* is to give the control group something that they think is reflexology but does not have the same effect or significance. Here, in my experience, is a really difficult problem. One way would be to randomly select people who had never even heard of reflexology and who, therefore, would not know what to expect and, more importantly, would not feel left out or cheated of a genuine treatment. But as reflexology has become known more widely, this is becoming more difficult, if not impossible. If the problem of a suitable substitute 'treatment' can be overcome, we have a *patient-blinded placebo – randomised control trial* and that is about as good as it gets for therapies like reflexology. I confess that, at the time of writing, I know of no substitute treatment that would withstand rigorous constructive criticism of its validity. To apply the therapy to inappropriate points on the foot for the condition presented – as in Olson and Flacco's study of 35 women with premenstrual symptoms – is to introduce a distortion. Our present knowledge leads us to believe that treating the 'wrong points' would not benefit the patient. But if it enhanced circulation and, as a consequence the health of tissue cells, who can say what benefit would be enjoyed and what impact that would have had on, for example, the premenstrual syndrome of Olsen and Flacco's study.

The Randomised Control Trial (RCT) within a well-defined protocol appears to have the widest valid application for reflexology. After all, it is regarded as the 'gold standard' test of the efficacy of medical treatments and a great deal is made of the need for evidence-based medicine.

One thing remains clear. Designing research studies that are capable of withstanding scientific (or do we mean objective?) scrutiny requires a great amount of time, effort and collaboration between practitioners and researchers and, above all, the financial support and perseverance to see it through to an outcome that has significance and value.

Research that nit-picks as it challenges that of which there is much anecdotal evidence stretching back over thousands of years (not necessarily in the Western world) adds very little. Neither is it of value or interest to increasing numbers of the public who know already that they feel healthier as a consequence of the therapy received. Research that extends the boundaries of our knowledge and, as a consequence, leads to or contributes towards a cure of chronic or life-threatening disease is truly justifiable and should receive all the collective support and encouragement it is in our power to give.

Basic Requirements of a Research Project

A first step in a research project is the design and clarification of its description or protocol. It is important to spend time and effort at this stage – which can be at odds with our natural enthusiasm to get started.

The protocol has two prime purposes:

1. It forms the basis of any submission for financial support.
2. It acts as the working schedule of the project.

Consequently, it is a great advantage if the protocol is as clear and unambiguous as possible. The competition for finance can be intense and only the best-formulated projects win support.

To assist those directly involved in the project (the project group) it helps to have the whole project in outline plan and written down; this keeps us focused. It is too easy to allow curiosity, enthusiasm or an unexpected 'discovery' or insight to divert us from our aim and / or to cause us to go over budget.

For a project to attract public support or research foundation support, the protocol must satisfy certain criteria and these are outlined below:

1. The background to the project is outlined. Existing research upon which our hypotheses are built are acknowledged and the relevance of the current research subject is discussed. Checking existing research is necessary to find out what the outcome was and it is a good idea to check the literature referenced in one or more databases. So, for reflexology, check what is held by The Association of Reflexologists, or Reflexology in Europe Network (see Useful Addresses), particularly the work done in Denmark, for example. Also, check what exists in China, the Far East and the USA. In the UK, check with the universities, for example, the Department of Complementary Medicine, Exeter. Similarly, Lancaster, Southampton, Westminster and Manchester.

2. The type of project. For reflexology, the RCT probably is the most suitable because, as with any touch therapy, the *Double Blind Randomised Control Trial* (DBRCT) is very difficult to apply in practice. Because it is difficult this does not mean, however, that we should not consider it.

3. The project's problems or limits are presented clearly. This can be thought of as a statement of what the project does not set out to verify or explore. More particularly, it can be a hypothesis that we wish to validate, for example. In reflexology work, this would be the stage where we would specify the type of therapy used (*see* page 125).

4. If a particular disease or symptom is involved, for example, the efficacy of reflexology therapy in alleviating symptoms of Irritable Bowel Syndrome (IBS) then the symptoms must be stated clearly. These form the criteria against which outcome, time and cost might be measured. In addition, who or what is to be included in the study or excluded from it? For example, what are to be the age limits of those patients within the study group, etc? What medication is being taken by those studied? Or, are we going to confine it to those not on prescribed medication? How will we cope if the medication is changed whilst the study is in progress? Or would this exclude them? These are the types of criteria we need to address and be clear about from the beginning. There are, of course, others but these should spark ideas.

5. The method of applied research is defined and described in detail to include a statement of the theories at the outset and which facts are accepted and taken for granted.

6. A statement of the method/s of data collection; questionnaires, interviews, blood samples, objective measurements (blood pressure, for example), video recording. Certain standard questionnaires exist and one that has achieved quite widespread credence is Measure Your Own Medical Outcome Profile (MYMOP) designed by Dr. Charlotte Patterson (with whom I had the privilege of working in a general medical practice, in Somerset, UK, in the early 1990s). As implied by its title, it involves the voluntary agreement and participation by a group of patients of sufficient number as to be significant and over a specified period of time.

7. Presentation of the parameters we are going to assess (e.g. blood pressure, pain on a defined scale of severity and / or type – dull, sharp, intermittent, variable, occasional (if so, how frequent?), etc., quality of life, mobility, etc. When studying the effects of reflexology treatments, remember to look at the parameters of possible side-effects.

8. A demonstration of how these theories, parameters and methods are relevant to the problem, disease, symptoms, hypothesis, we want to examine.

9. A discussion of how theories and methods influence the outcome of the study. What can or cannot be studied with the chosen methods?

10. A presentation of the written information to participating patients stating:

    • the purpose of the study;
    • the methods applied;
    • implications for individual participants;
    • that anyone can withdraw at any time;
    • that participation is entirely voluntary.

11. A discussion of the ethical implications for participants, e.g. confidentiality of both participation and outcome, voluntary (payments would distort) and guaranteed anonymity.

12. A list of researchers with their curriculum vitae, past research and published papers, together with a list of participating patients.

13. A description of how the outcome would be published and an indication of the scope, population, to whom it might apply or be of interest.

14. A detailed time schedule.

15. A detailed budget and rate at which funding would be used, i.e. a cash flow forecast.

16. The name of two project leaders (two to give cover) elected to be responsible for all aspects of the project and to whom all relevant matters should be addressed.

Useful Advice

It is not helpful to state, for example, that the purpose of the project is to prove that treatment X is successful. Instead, perhaps, write that the purpose is to study whether treatment X works according to specific chosen parameters, with continual assessment against those criteria during the course of the project.

Always adopt a detached (as much as this is possible) critical and investigative attitude towards the subject to be studied. A project confined to a 'one and only truth' would not receive the support of large foundations nor would the outcome have the respect of contemporary research establishments.

Frequently, the universities have academically trained people either out of a job or for whom undertaking research forms part of their training who may be available to help. Also, they can provide an unbiased, detached approach, with no direct influence or financial interest in the outcome.

Some Reference Material

I am indebted to Mr. Anthony Porter, Director of ART (*see* Useful Addresses) for the following summary of the techniques used by practicing reflexologists (*see* Appendix to Chapter 6). Originally, it was produced for the Reflexology Research Trust; the brainchild of Hazel Goodwin, past Chairman of the Association of Reflexologists (UK).

The brief, summarised work, researched in Denmark and in China are included in the Appendix for reference only. The Audit (see Appendix to Chapter 7), serves as a link with these studies and as a thread between this chapter and the next.

A Consideration of the Various Types of Reflex Contact for Comparison in Reflexology Research

It is imperative that the various types and techniques of reflexology used by reflexologists are recognised for their therapeutic value before it can be established which are to be used in a research programme.

Rather than discussing the various teaching organisations of these techniques, it was decided to simplify the matter by listing the procedures themselves. For this purpose, listed below are the main types of contact; there may well be others which fall outside these spheres.

Ingham Method
This forms the basis of Western reflexological practice. It is a very specific method of what is best described as finger and thumb walking on all the areas of the feet. Combined with this is a range of methods of providing support and control for the hands and feet while these various contacts are being made. The Ingham method (copyright) is the technique which was formulated by Eunice Ingham, who was known as the 'Mother' of reflexology in the 1930s. This technique is only (officially) taught by The International Institute of Reflexology. Used properly, it is a very effective form of reflexology which promotes a firm and positive contact. This 'finger and thumb' walking method is the most common technique in use, particularly in the Western world. Unfortunately, the key principles of this method have become diluted by misguided tuition from teaching schools outside the I.I.R.

Light Touch Techniques
Pioneered by Patricia Morrell, and as the name implies, the contact is very light and gentle. The recipient feels no discomfort from the 'disturbed' reflexes. This technique has enjoyed considerable success in the post-operative treatment of orthopaedic conditions such as hip and knee replacement.

Linking
This is another light touch technique which applies contact to two or more reflex points at once using *constant* light pressure as distinct from the more orthodox finger and thumb moving technique. It is a very relaxing type of approach. Recipients of this therapy often feel a sensation of warmth in the corresponding reflex areas being treated.

Energetic Reflexology
This type of reflexology (if it can be called reflexology) is well-known in Israel and to an extent in Germany. There is no physical contact to the feet – the hands being held close to the skin which are sometimes static and sometimes making slow movements around the feet.

Vertical Reflex Reflexology (VRT)
This technique, developed by Lynne Booth, is a unique way of treating orthopaedic conditions such as lower back problems, knee and hip conditions. Through development, conditions other than those mentioned are becoming responsive to the technique. It is unique because the patient is treated while standing up.

It is this vertical weight-bearing position that seems to amplify the reflex situation. The treatment is short and intense lasting about five minutes. Initial evidence is showing VRT to be highly effective. Controlled trials are underway, and those who have experienced this treatment have found it very therapeutic, particularly lower back problems.

Positive / Dynamic Techniques of Reflexology

This type of reflex contact, performed by an adequately trained reflexologist, can bring about strong therapeutic reactions. This type of treatment can be used with the more orthodox finger / thumb walking, by giving a deeper contact to the reflexes. Some of the Far Eastern practitioners use special types of reflexology sticks to make a deep and concentrated contact to the reflexes, while others will use the knuckles. To perform these types of techniques a lubricant is used on the feet.

A vast amount of reflexology being used today is not what can be called *clinical* reflexology. This is because of the varying standards of teaching, and the lack of understanding and experience by many teachers. It often means that in many instances, reflexology sometimes at best is nothing more than a light foot massage.

Experience indicates that a positive and concentrated contact (where appropriate) to the reflexes generally produces quicker therapeutic responses than a light contact.

Advanced Reflexology Treatment (ART)

This treatment uses a number of techniques which include a positive and sometimes concentrated contact. Anecdotal evidence is showing that using a combination of these techniques is producing a great deal of patient satisfaction, particularly in the treatment of various gynaecological conditions.

Methodology of Research Considerations

The usually accepted treatment programme is once a week. For a general treatment this is satisfactory, but a clinical treatment for a specific condition this programme would not be satisfactory and as the research will probably be based on the treatment of clinical conditions, different treatment programmes will have to be considered.

Clinical reflexology can be carried out by an experienced and properly trained therapist on a *daily* basis, i.e. five days, then two days off, four days the following week then three days, before reviewing the treatment results. With this mode of treatment the duration should not exceed half an hour; sometimes 15–20 minutes is enough.

Researchers' Requirements

It is vital that those taking part in the research have been in full-time practice for at least five years. The term 'full-time' also has to be defined. For instance, a practitioner could be in full-time practice, yet only treat 5 patients weekly. Also, what type of treatment are they used to giving; clinical or general?

The ideal researcher would be one who has been in practice for the duration as defined, gives a minimum of 15 treatments weekly, and is used to giving clinical treatments. Ideally, they should be experienced in all aspects and styles of reflexology.

Chapter 7

Treating Stroke Patients

A group of patients that deserve our utmost sympathy and understanding are those who have suffered a debilitating stroke. In a split second, their life has been turned upside down. At the snap of your fingers just imagine that you no longer have use of half your body, your speech may be lost or severely impaired, you don't even know if you are upright, leaning sideways, backwards or forward; you have lost all spatial awareness. It is easy to see how the word 'stroke' comes from the Old English for 'blow; or 'calamity'.

The shock to the constitution can compare only to the sufferer's shattered morale. This is why we must respect their predicament and work hard to get them mobile and to restore the best quality of life that is possible.

Their mood swings, during the long recovery process, are more extreme than for those of us who remain healthy. It is important, therefore, to give realistic encouragement and never to say that, because a particular period of time has past since the stroke, they cannot expect any further significant improvement. My experience is that such an opinion is not only false but it is demoralising to the person. How can even the most eminent consultant know the degree to which the body is capable of healing itself? It remains one of the most fascinating unknowns of the health care world.

Strokes can happen to those who are 'in charge' – whether by job title or of a personality that likes to be in charge of others and events. They can, of course, happen to any one of us, but others have observed a tendency, they claim, to 'in-charge' types. Statistically, a fifth of all stroke victims in the UK are under the age of 40. We can use these figures another way; 80% of stroke victims are beyond the age of 40 – so under 40's don't get too anxious.

Strokes, known as brain attacks in the USA, affecting the left side of the brain and causing right-side hemiplegia and loss of speech is perhaps the most frustrating for the patient. To listen and to be bursting to reply or join in a conversation (to think the words) yet be unable to speak them must be very hard to bear.

Recovery from left-sided hemiplegia requires learning all over again; to put one foot in front of the other. Similarly, patients recovering from right-sided hemiplegia have to learn to put one word in front of the next. Each 'step' takes an enormous amount of will power and determination.

Consequently, any patient will, at times, feel that they will never recover and this leads to periods of deep depression and anger. Some of the emotional aspects of stroke recovery are listed (*see* page 137).

To avoid repetition and to provide a comprehensive reference, the following Audit (*see* Appendix to Chapter 7) covers many of the aspects of a stroke recovery programme.

I remain utterly convinced of the value of cautious optimism in our encouragement and support of patients; whilst helping them to accept that the recovery programme will be long and, at times, arduous. Their determination, patience, constitutional powers of recovery and the continued support and encouragement of immediate family and friends are paramount.

A Definition

Damage to part of the brain caused by an interruption of the blood supply to it or by leakage of blood through the walls of blood vessels in it.

Introduction

The brain is highly sensitive to even temporary ischemia and if the oxygen loss in the tissues (anoxia) is severe or total, nerve cells are damaged beyond repair. In just a few minutes the nerves of the cortex of the cerebellum can be affected.

At the beginning of my work with stroke patients, I had not appreciated that the brain's main 'food' is glucose, which is carried in the carotid arteries' blood supply to the brain. Glucose enables the cerebral neurons to store and then secrete the messenger chemicals; the *neurotransmitters* and *neuropeptides*. It also energises the glial cells within the brain; these are neural cells that have a connective tissue supporting function in the central nervous system. These glial cells act in a similar way to the macrophages of the immune system – peptide 'cleaners' that move around, sometimes destroying and sometimes nurturing nerve-endings. Only when there is a sufficient blood flow to supply the brain with glucose and oxygen can the neurons and glial cells function properly.

I well remember being asked to treat a patient, by his wife, whilst he was in the first 48 hours of hospitalisation, following a severe stroke. During the necessary courtesy of getting clearance to go on to the ward, it was assumed that the patient was on Warfarin and / or Heparin (both anticoagulants) only to be told by the consultant, somewhat curtly, that he was receiving glucose.

On the first visit, at which the nursing staff made his medical notes available to me, the severity of his condition was obvious. The glucose was being given intravenously as the patient was slipping in and out of consciousness. When, subsequently, full consciousness was restored, the glucose supply was ceased. It is a point of conjecture whether continuation of a glucose supplemented diet would have been of additional help to him, or indeed other patients.

There are two major factors affecting the amount of blood reaching the brain:

1. The condition of the heart and its ability to pump efficiently, and;
2. the condition of the arteries.

The amount of oxygen and other nutrients in the blood and the 'stickiness' (viscosity) of the blood can also have an influence upon good quality blood supply to the brain.

A simple faint (syncope) is a temporary suspension of consciousness due to generalized cerebral ischemia so brief as to cause no lasting structural damage.

Transient Ischaemic Attacks (TIAs), are similar and can be due to partial, temporary occlusion of the carotid arteries. The symptoms last less than 24 hours and are a warning of insufficient blood reaching the brain.

Types of Stroke

Cerebral Thrombosis ('Static' Clot)
This type accounts for approximately 45% of cases. Leads to cessation of blood supply to part of the brain by a clot (thrombosis) that has adhered to and built up on the wall of an artery in the brain. Causes infarction; tissue death due to oxygen and cell-nutritional starvation.

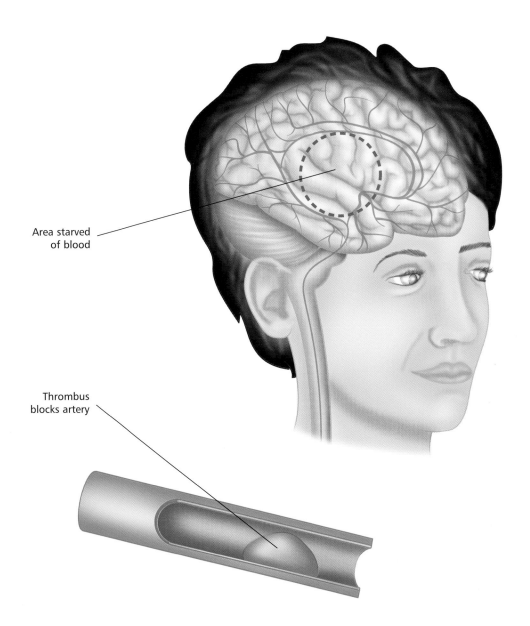

Area starved
of blood

Thrombus
blocks artery

Figure 7/1: Cerebral thrombosis.

Cerebral Embolism ('Mobile' Clot)
Similarly, the blood supply can be blocked by an embolus travelling in an artery until it reaches a point where it cuts off the blood flow. Again, this causes localised tissue death. Accounts for approximately 32% of strokes.

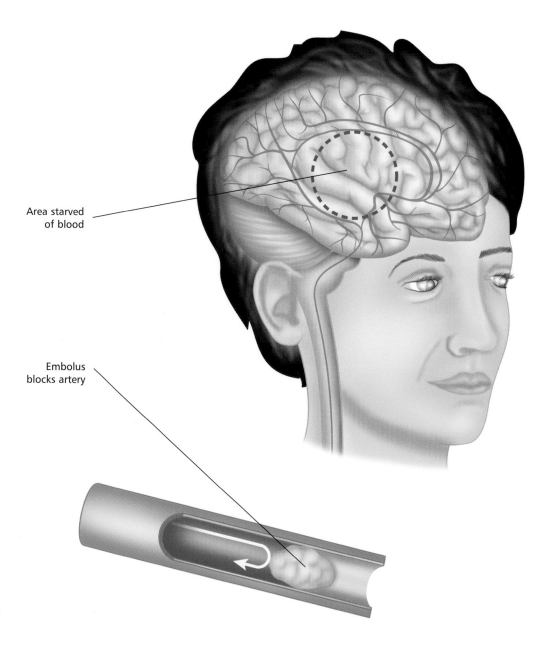

Area starved
of blood

Embolus
blocks artery

*Figure 7/2: Cerebral
embolism.*

Haemorrhage
This is the consequence of the rupture of a blood vessel leading to bleeding within or over the surface of the brain, and is the cause in approximately 23% of strokes.

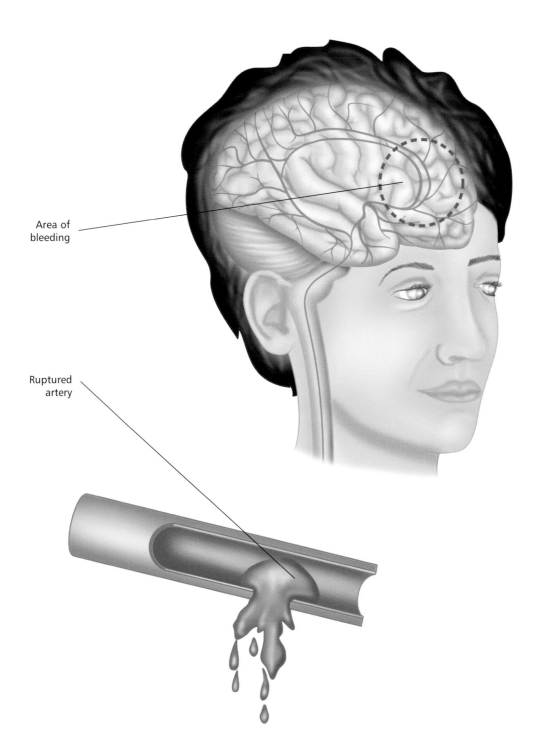

Area of
bleeding

Ruptured
artery

Figure 7/3:
Haemorrhage.

Pathological appearance of a stroke shows up on a Magnetic Resonance Image (MRI) or on a photograph (X-ray) as a dark area, indicating bleeding and starvation of oxygen in that area.

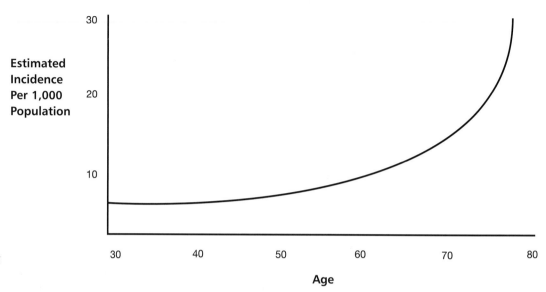

Figure 7/4:
Incidence of strokes
in relation to age.

In the UK, the overall number of strokes is about 200 per 100,000 population per year (.02%). The incidence rises steeply with age (as shown above) and it is higher in men than in women.

Probable contributing factors that may increase the chances of suffering a stroke are:

• High blood pressure (hypertension) which puts extra strain on the walls of the arteries.
• Narrowing of arteries (atherosclerosis) – by fatty deposits.
• Heart beat irregularity (atrial fibrillation)   Can lead to blood clots in the
• Damaged heart valve or malfunctioning valve   heart that may break away and
• Recent heart attack (myocardial infarction)   find their way into the brain.
• High levels of fatty substances in the blood (hyperlipidaemia).
• Diabetes mellitus and smoking can also increase the risk by increasing the chances of hypertension and atherosclerosis.

All of the above factors can be reduced or influenced by a nutritious diet, reduction of stress, regular physical exercise and plenty of pure water and fresh air. Equally, it could be argued that a similar lifestyle provides us with the best chance of avoiding ailments generally.

Signs and Symptoms

We know that sensation and movement on one side of the body is controlled by the cerebral hemisphere on the opposite side. Hence, damage to the right cerebral hemisphere causes loss of sensation and movement of the left side of the body. Because the control for speech is in the left cerebral hemisphere, those who are left-side affected by a stroke in the right side of the brain usually retain the power of speech which can be slurred at first because of the one-sided paralysis of vocal cords, tongue, lips and mouth. Often a facial sign of a stroke is that the mouth drops on one side.

One sided weakness or paralysis of the body is called *hemiplegia* and disturbance of speech is called *aphasia*.

In general, damage to a specific area of the brain from a stroke (or injury) impairs bodily sensation, movement or function controlled by that part of the brain.

Summary of Signs and Symptoms of a Stroke – Onset

- Headache
- Dizziness and confusion ⎫ may be just pre-
- Visual disturbance ⎬ or at onset
- Loss of speech or slurred speech
- Difficulty swallowing (dysphagia)

Whilst the symptoms of a stroke can occur over several days, it is more likely that they develop abruptly and quite unexpectedly over minutes or hours.

Depending on the location, cause and extent of damage, any or all of the symptoms listed above may be present in any degree of severity.

Severe cases involve loss of consciousness and can progress to coma and death. Alternatively, the patient may have severe physical or mental handicap. At the other end of the spectrum of outcome, a stroke can be so mild as to cause symptoms that are barely noticeable, e.g. a slight limp when walking.

Approximately a third of major strokes are fatal; a third leave disability and a third have no apparent lasting effects.

Post-stroke Emotions

The careful observation of my patients over a significant period of time has lead to the following conclusion regarding the emotional changes (mood swings), that patients can experience.

- Disbelief
- Shock
- Fear
- Anger
- Despair
- Frustration
- Depression
- Loneliness
- Worthlessness

Post-stroke Recovery Qualities

- Constitutional health
- Determination
- Courage

- Patience
- Perseverance
- Self-reconciliation
- Self-belief

Assisted by (a 'blended mix' is needed to achieve best patient-help):

- Mainstream medicine
- Physiotherapy
- Occupational therapy
- Complementary therapy

It can be argued that the same pre- and post-emotional symptoms apply to all patients who have suffered the misfortune of a severe illness. But, in my experience, these symptoms are much more sharply pronounced in stroke sufferers – it is as if they are proportional to the sudden and severe shock of the occurrence, the instant nature of it. One can only imagine that a war wound or a severe motor accident also having a similar instant adverse shock-impact upon the body's physical and emotional wellbeing.

Appendix to Chapter 6

Research Data

Research – Denmark

The Department of Social Pharmacy, The Royal Danish School of Pharmacy, in co-operation with 5 reflexology societies completed a 3 month survey on the treatment of 200 patients with *migraine and tension headaches*.

Outcome (initially): Effective in 78% of all patients, of whom 23% claimed 'cure' and 55% claimed to be 'helped'.

Outcome (follow-up, 3 months later): 16% reported being 'cured'; 65% reported being helped; 18% reported no change; 1% failed to report.

Reference

Reflexions, **42**, *International Journal of Alternative & Complementary Med.*, May 1996.

Research – China

A recent analysis of 8096 clinical cases by Dr. Wang Liang reported in the 1996 China Reflexology Symposium Report of the China Reflexology Association found foot reflexology to be 93.63% effective in treating 63 disorders.

Dr. Liang found that foot reflexology proved to be: significantly effective (cure) in 48.68% of all cases; effective or improvement in 44.95%; no effect in 6.37%.

Dr. Liang found foot reflexolgoy to be: 100% effective in treating 7 disorders; 90% effective for 45 of the disorders; significantly effective 50% or more of the time for 22 disorders.

Criteria for Evaluation

The criteria for evaluation of clinical effect followed the 3 grades typical of modern medicine:

1. Cure or significantly effective: *"A disease disappears or does not recur in a relatively long time."*

2. Improvement or effective: *"Most of the symptoms disappear or partly disappear and the patient feels the symptoms are ameliorated and markedly improved ... if treatment stopped, the original symptoms and signs may recur."*

3. No effect or ineffective: *"There is no improvement of the symptoms and signs of a disease or, the improvement is very insignificant".*

Reference

Liang, Wang. (1996). *An exploration of the Clinical Indication of Foot Reflexology, A Retrospective Analysis of Its Clinical Application of 8096 Cases*. China Reflexology Symposium Report. China Reflexology Association, October 1996, Beijing.

Appendix to Chapter 7

An Audit of the Contribution of Reflexology to Stroke Recovery Programmes

Purpose

Primary: To audit, in measured terms (i.e. *quantitative*), the recovery of a number of post stroke patients who had received reflexology treatment as part of, or complementary to, the programme used within mainstream medicine.

Secondary: To alert those whom it concerns to consider the possible benefits of including reflexology when designing a post-stroke recovery programme.

Introduction

1. Significant statistics.
2. A definition of a stroke.

1. Significant Statistics

- Over 12,500 stroke victims die or are left disabled because of lack of specialist care.
- Only one in three spent any time in a specialist unit.
- Only just over half spent the majority of their hospital stay in a specialist unit.
- Strokes are UK's third biggest killer – approximately 130,000 people suffer an attack each year and increasing.
- Research shows: 19% of patients saved by treatment in stroke units; and 29% of survivors avoid becoming dependent on carers.
- From 1999–2001/2: One patient in five did not get a brain scan.
- One in ten did not receive drugs they should have been prescribed on leaving hospital.
- Four out of five (80%) hospitals now have a stroke specialist working approximately 8 hours per week – equivalent to 33 full time doctors in England and Wales. Should be 418 (say 'experts').
- Government's target of specialist stroke units in all hospitals by 2004 unlikely to be achieved (source: Royal College of Physicians article, Jenny Hope, *Daily Mail* (24/07/02)).

2. A Definition of a Stroke

Damage to part of the brain caused by an interruption of the blood supply to it or by leakage of blood through the walls of blood vessels in it.

Extracts From Four Case Studies

- Personal details
- Occupation
- Medical history
- Medication, including Adverse Drug Reaction/s (ADR's)
- When first seen by reflexologist
- Presenting signs / symptoms / information
- Tender areas of feet at initial consultation
- Presenting indications re. the above
- Patient's aim
- Therapist's aim
- Significant events in treatment outcome
- Summary of outcome

Graphical Data

The above is supported by the case studies; graphs, i.e. measured movement (inches above horizontal) of hitherto paralysed leg, plotted against time (days after stroke).

Some Overall Results

All patients were treated on the feet, using the Ingham Method; that is firm pressure most of the time (pressure is varied to suit the condition, health and age of patient presented).

- Patient A had 44 treatments spread over 636 days.
- Patient B had 71 treatments spread over 625 days.
- Patient C had 22 treatments spread over 298 days.
- Patient D had 68 treatments spread over 368 days.

There was some suggested commonality of areas found to be tender or very tender at the outset. But the sample is too small to form any valid conclusions. For the record, the most common tender areas at the outset were: eyes; kidneys; ears; parietal area of brain; sinuses (facial); thyroid; adrenals (75% of sample); spine; pancreas; pituitary; ileocaecal valve.

The above broadly suggests the endocrine, digestive and cranial nerves as the body systems that may be most affected, with the urinary system as 'secondary' influence.

Stroke Patient Case Studies (Patient 'A')

Personal Details   Male, height 5'10" (1.78m), weight 18 stone (114.3kg).

Occupation   Retired farmer.

Medical History   Age, at time of stroke, 60 years.

Subarachnoid haemorrhage 2 years, 2 months before first seen. Initially, admitted to Frenchay Hospital, Bristol, and emergency surgery done, followed by Intensive Care Unit (ICU) and rehabilitation at the Bristol Royal Infirmary (BRI) (both UK).

• Suffered post-stroke, occasional epilepsy.
• Took first steps (calliper supported) 14 months before first seen.
• Total paralysis of left arm, limited range of movement of left leg.
• Speech – slightly slurred.

N.B. Unquenchable appetite – as if stomach without sensation of feeling full.
Non-smoker; non-diabetic; moderate alcohol intake per week (prior to stroke).

Medication

1. Tegretol (carbamazepine) 200mg (2bd).
   Function: analgesic and anti convulsant (re. tendency to epilepsy).
   ADR's: dizziness and gastro-intestinal disturbance.

2. Adalat Retard (nifedipine).
   Function: calcium channel-blocking vasodilator.
   ADR's: flushing (present); headache; ankle oedema (present).

First Seen

2 years, 2 months after the stroke, i.e. when patient was 62 years+.

Presenting Signs / Symptoms / Information

• Patient and wife agreed he suffered from flatus.
• Reduced vision of left eye, post stroke.
• Patient reported some spinal pain and general discomfort.
• Patient quoted 'nervous tummy', i.e. bouts of diarrhoea (Tegretol ADR).
• Left arm, no sensation or movement.
• Left leg, some voluntary movement but impaired motor control.
• Patient looked overweight and flushed (ref. Adalat Retard ADR) and ankle oedema (left and right) was present (ref. Adalat Retard ADR).

Tender Areas of Feet at Initial Consultation (2 years, 2 months after stroke)

- Left and right ears and eyes and middle ear area.
- Sinuses (frontal and maxillary).
- Gallbladder.
- Adrenals, pituitary and tail of pancreas.
- Ileocaceal valve and sigmoid flexure.
- Kidneys.
- Right parietal area of brain (site of haemorrhage and subsequent surgery).

Presenting Indications re. the Above

Possible ENT weakness and tendency to occasional dizziness and 'thick heads'. Probable intolerance to foods of high fat-content. Low constitutional energy and tendency to digestive problems. Suspected lack of normal bowel function.

The patient and his wife confirmed the accuracy of the above, indicated by an initial reflexology 'exploration' of the feet and ankles.

Patient's Aim

To regain full mobility and independence.

Therapist's Aim

To achieve as much recovery of mobility of which the patient's constitution is capable, plus to boost the patient's morale – to restore the ability to enjoy life again within the confines of some loss of function / sensation.

Significant Events in Treatment Outcome

At 3rd treatment (14 days after 1st)	Patient reported tingling ('pins and needles') sensation in left heel.
4th (21 days)	Left leg felt less 'heavy' (patient quote).
5th (28 days)	With OT, patient had walked without walking stick and OT commented that patient's muscles were working better – more co-ordinated.
6th (35 days)	Patient had experienced more energy and increased mental alertness – less tendency to doze during daytime.
9th (49 days)	Patient had walked to toilet, holding on to wheelchair (approx. 18 metres on level floor).
10th (56 days)	Momentary left leg lift, whilst seated, of 10in. (25.5cm) vertically (measured at heel). Patient could flex left leg and knee. Left leg lift, progress as shown on graph.
18th (97 days)	Patient asked to see if left knee would lift; achieved a 'tremor' movement of 1/2in. (13mm) vertically.

20th (111 days)	Left arm felt 'lighter' (patient quote).
21st (118 days)	Left knee lift 2in. (5cm) vertically.
23rd (132 days)	Noticed that patient could speak coherently and clearly forapproximately 45 minutes, **without fatigue**. Left leg lift, as shown on graph.
27th (153 days)	Patient had not practised his physio. / OT's exercises. Lack of willpower apparent.
38th (461 days)	Patient tense (not exercising) patient 'bullied' into action to prevent losing good work of physio., OT and reflexology. Patient joined indoor bowls club and a social club (social life again)!
41st (552 days)	Two weeks residential respite – no exercise, plus a fall, set patient's mobility and morale back and reduced confidence to move about.
42nd (580 days)	Fluid build-up: kidney reflex areas very tender. Patient 'plateaued'; he lost incentive and seemed to settle for what he had.
44th (636 days)	He was no longer prepared to work at improving himself. The respite period seemed to have had a lasting adverse effect.

Summary Outcome

• Clarity, duration and coherence of speech improved (to 45 minutes without fatigue).

• Left leg ability to lift vertically, whilst sat, improved and thereby muscle strength increased.

• Hope, plus positive self-evidence of a degree of physical improvement boosted morale.

• To an extent, a proportion of the above progress was negated during respite period.

• Consequently, patient settled for what he had and, in my view, had become tired of our 'encouragement' to strive for any possible further improvement.

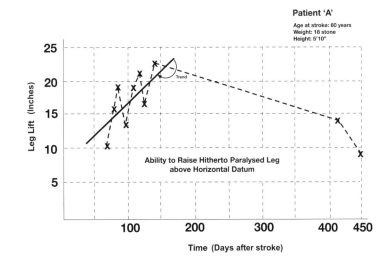

Patient 'A'

Age at stroke: 60 years
Weight: 18 stone
Height: 5'10"

Leg Lift (Inches)

Ability to Raise Hitherto Paralysed Leg above Horizontal Datum

Time (Days after stroke)

Stroke Patient Case Studies (Patient 'B')

Personal Details	Male, height 5'10½" (1.78m), weight 11st 2lb (70kg).
Occupation	HGV driver.
Medical History	Age, at time of stroke, 52 years, 8 months.

Previously of good general health. A worrier, quick tempered and holds some very definite opinions bordering on perfection.

Admitted to hospital with cerebral thrombosis of right temporal area, resulting from an almost complete occlusion of his right carotid artery.

Left side hemiplegia – i.e. complete paralysis of left side of body and affected throat and pharyngeal area such that patient was fed via a glucose drip. His balance and righting reactions were impaired to the extent that, after initial bed rest, he was unable to sit unaided. Indeed, he had no concept of 'where he was'. He required full nursing care and the hospital prognosis doubted his ability to return home.

At onset, patient was aware of a headache, with blurred vision and pain radiating from frontal to occipital area.

Medication

1. Epilim 200mg (tbs), 300mg (2bd) (sodium valproate).
   Function: anti convulsant and anti epileptic.
   ADR's: nausea and gastric irritation; unsteady gait and muscle tremor; increased appetite and weight gain; temporary hair loss, oedema, blood changes, impaired liver function, rashes, growth of breasts in men!
   Warning: should not be administered to patients with liver disease or family history of liver dysfunction (would the patient know this?!). Administer with caution to patients who are pregnant or breast feeding, or who have lupus erythematosus.

2. Aspirin (tbs) (acetylsalicylic acid); 75mg (1bd).
   Function: NSAID, non-narcotic analgesic and anti-rheumatic and anti-pyretic (temperature-reducer) for colds and fevers. At low dosage acts as anti-platelet treatment for those at risk.
   ADR's: gastrointestinal upsets, dyspepsia (indigestion), nausea, diarrhoea, bleeding and ulceration. May be hypersensitivity reactions; including rash, bronchospasm, oedema, headache, blood disorders, ringing in the ears and fluid retention. Gastrointestinal reaction can be minimised by taking drug with milk or food.

First Seen

In hospital 3 days after stroke, i.e. on Monday afternoon; stroke occurred on the previous Saturday morning.

Presenting Signs / Symptoms / Information

- Patient confined to bed and quite seriously ill.
- Drifted in and out of sleep / consciousness.
- Dysplasia (difficulty in swallowing) – no sensation of tongue, mouth, throat, etc.

Tender Areas of Feet at Initial Consultation

Little 'reaction' because of patient's condition. But, tender spot on right side of brain area, coincident with site of thrombus. Worked on: shoulders, cervicals, whole spine and diaphragm and diaphragm relaxant. (Patient had good cough soon after treating this area).

Therapist's Aim

To recover as much mobility and return to normal health as possible – over a long period of time.

Significant Events in Treatment Outcome

1st treatment (3 days after stroke)	Immediately post treatment (deliberately brief) whole of left hallux and areas of cervicals and upper thoracic area turned an inflamed red colour. Patient murmured that treatment "felt great".
2nd treatment	Patient had good night's sleep after first treatment plus increased control of swallowing.
3rd (18 days)	Patient transferred to rehab. unit. Physio. sessions mornings and afternoons (approximately 1 hour sessions). Brief reflexology treatment (patient very tired).

That evening, patient moved toes of left foot very slightly and voluntarily; able to repeat movement at will for observing visiting family members.

4th (25 days)	Patient raised left leg (at heel) 5in. (13cm) above horizontal bed surface and 'bent' knee to 2/3in. (2cm) above horizontal.
6th (39 days)	Patient's face had more normal appearance. **Patient can stand unsupported for about 10 seconds** (physios. doing a wonderful job).
7th (46 days)	**Patient stood, unaided, from sitting position** during observed physiotherapy session.

– Patient returned home –

9th (74 days)	Left leg raised 9in. (23cm) above horizontal (patient seated).
10th (81 days)	Patient moved left thumb and had sensory sensation in left shoulder.
15th (117 days)	Patient had, what he called, bad spell (gets these every 6/7 weeks) paralysis returns to facial muscles and loss of sensation of where food is in the mouth.
16th (124 days)	Patient raised left arm, against gravity, to 90° elbow bend, forearm straight.
17th (132 days)	Patient can get into and out of bath. Left leg raised 10 1/2in. (26cm) above horizontal.

19th (144 days)	Patient had done a lot of walking and exercise (up and down stairs, etc.) **Bed going back upstairs next week.**
22nd (174 days)	Patient despondent – physio. treatment no longer so attentive or advantageous or challenging.

– left leg raising increased progressively, as shown on graph –

36th (272 days)	Patient can grip with left hand, but cannot release grip.
38th (293 days)	Patient had epileptic attack 3 days after previous treatment. Doctor prescribed Epilim 150mg (2bd).
39th (301 days)	Patient calm and confidence has not suffered.
47th (385 days)	Left leg raised to a maximum 27in. (68.5cm) above horizontal! **Now getting patient to hold leg up** (achieved 14in. (35.5cm) for 4 seconds).
54th (488 days)	Patient depressed – useless lower leg support made – won't wear it. Medical notes not transferred between hospitals.
70th (618 days)	Leg lift, kick action, to 36in. (91.5cm) above horizontal. Patient held leg at 12–14in. (30.5–35.5cm) above horizontal for 25 seconds. **Left hand can do pincer movement with forefinger and thumb.**
71st (625 days)	Patient in good health and spirits, walking further, in co-ordinated, careful way, swings leg and stamina increasing steadily.

Summary Outcome

- Epileptic attacks infrequent, 2 in 3 years, second far less severe.

- Increasing stamina enabled patient to walk over one mile and to be on feet for half-day periods.

- Constitutionally, appears healthy.

- Gets lonely, with proportional depression, occasionally.

- Wife no longer able to cope, after giving initial 100% help and encouragement, and separated from patient after 3$\frac{1}{2}$ years of stroke.

- Patient in respite care for 2 weeks, following separation, then allowed to return home to "give it a go" (quote).

- Patient has proved he can cope (6 weeks after separation) and is dealing with divorce and house sale without any signs of regression, i.e. he is self-sufficient 3$\frac{1}{2}$ years after stroke.

Note: Subsequently this man regained his driving licence (for an adapted vehicle). This was a very significant event. He also learned to ride a horse and won prizes on it (he had never ridden before in his life).

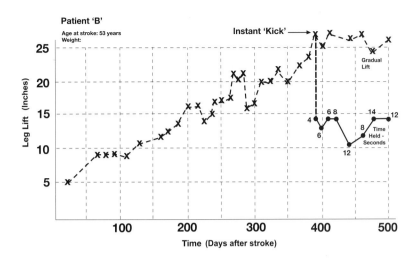

Stroke Patient Case Studies (Patient 'C')

Personal Details	Male, height 6'1" (1.85m), weight 15 stone (95.25kg).
Occupation	Retired.
Medical History	Age, at time of stroke, 73 years. Stroke paralysed whole of left side and, for two weeks, affected speech. Patient right-handed.

Non-smoker; non-diabetic; very moderate alcohol per week (prior to stroke). Physiotherapy and OT ceased approximately 2 years after stroke.

Medication

1. Digoxin 5mg, at night.
   Function: atrial fibrillation; supraventricular tachycardia, heart failure.
   Drug enhances calcium entry into cells; enhancing cardiac contraction and prolonged refractory period of atrioventricular (AV) node.
   Cautions: hypokalaemia, hypothyroidism, recent myocardial infarction, renal impairment, elderly.
   Contraindication: Wolff-Parkinson-White syndrome.
   ADR's: anorexia, fatigue, nausea and vomiting, abdominal pain, visual disturbances, anhythmias and heart block.
   Interactions: Increased blood levels with: Verapamil, Nifedipine, Amiodarone, and Quinidine.
   Increased toxicity with hypokalaemia.
   Increased risk AV block with beta-blockers, Verapamil.

2. Celevac (methylcellose, laxative bulking agent) 500mg (4 bd).
   Function: Increases overall mass of faeces and retains water, so stimulating bowel action.
   Can be used in patients with bran intolerance.
   Limitations: Full effect may not be for many hours. **Must not be administered to patients with intestinal obstruction**, lack of colon tone or faecal impaction. Fluid intake during treatment should be higher than usual.
   Should not be taken last thing at night.
   ADR's are mild and include flatulence, abdominal distension, faecal impaction and lack of tone in the colon.

3. Ditropan (oxybutynin hydrochloride) 5mg, at night.
   Function: Anticholinergic. Can be used as an antispasmodic in treating urinary frequency and incontinence.
   ADR's: dry mouth, blurred vision, constipation, nausea, abdominal discomfort, difficulty in urination, flushing of face, headache, dizziness, diarrhoea, dry skin and heart irregularities.
   Warning: Should not be administered to patients with: intestinal obstruction, severe ulcerative colitis, toxic megacolon, glaucoma or bladder obstruction.
   Care needed with patients who have certain heart, liver or kidney disorders, hyperthyroidism, prostatic hypertrophy, hiatus hernia with reflux oesophagitis or who are pregnant or breast-feeding.

First Seen

6 years after stroke.

Presenting Signs / Symptoms / Information

Patient, in his younger years, was a keep top-class racing cyclist. Determination, typical of top competitors, was obvious. But it brings with it frustration – in this case, caused by dragging the left foot which scuffed the toecap of his left shoe. The left arm remained paralysed.

Tender Areas of Feet at Initial Consultation

Very tender areas: pituitary, thyroid, adrenals, spine (L1; T6/7, C5, C6/7), chronic medial rectum / sciatic groove, right shoulder (restricted physical movement).
Tender areas: ears / eyes, transverse colon, ileocaecal valve.

Presenting Indications re. the Above

Endocrine system below par and thyroid / adrenal tenderness indicated constitutional fatigue

Suffers back pain in which L1 may be influencing transverse colon condition / constipation (if any) etc. Suspicion of occasional dizziness (confirmed by patient – see also ADR's of medication). Problem with right shoulder.

Patient's Aim

To restore normal gait to left leg and thus avoid scuffing toecap of shoe.

Therapist's Aim

To re-balance constitution and to see to what extent paralysis could be alleviated – including the patient's declared aim.

Significant Events in Treatment Outcome

2nd (8 days after 1st)	For two days after first treatment had not felt as well 'generally' for years. This faded after 4 days.
3rd (14 days)	Left leg raised 10in. (25.5cm) above horizontal. Bad night after last treatment – diarrhoea; used to get it every other day but this was first bout in 14 days. Right shoulder remained very painful and had limited movement only.

4th (22 days)	Left leg lifted 8in. (20cm).
5th	Patient said "legs feel like jelly first thing in the morning and have done so since my stroke", i.e. for past 6 years.
8th (60 days)	Left leg raised 12in. (30.5cm).
9th (77 days)	Left leg raised 14in. (35.5cm) and 'pressure' experienced when urinating.
10th (91 days)	Left leg raised 15in. (38cm).
11th (112 days)	Left leg dragging again. Patient despondent.
12th (117 days)	Patient could close left index finger and thumb with enough strength and co-ordination to pick up a thin sheet of paper.
13th (129 days)	Patient feeling lethargic "could not care whether I live or die" and depressed state has lasted past 7/10 days. Out of character with personality displayed hitherto.
14th (143 days)	Left hip pain making walking difficult.
15th (157 days)	Left leg raised 17in. (43cm) – leg no longer drags. Patient asked therapist if it would be possible to gain movement back in left arm.
16th (171 days)	Patient had experienced severe chest pain (not radiated into left arm) approximately 7 days ago. Subsequent X-ray clear. Doctor re-prescribed Digoxin – to help breathing. **Shoulder more mobile; left arm swings when walking (no longer kept in left pocket all the time).**
17th (185 days)	Doctor reduced Digoxin which, overall, had produced an adverse effect upon patient. Patient advised to report ADR to doctor.
18th (199 days)	Patient looking healthier and in good spirits.
19th (208 days)	Patient in buoyant mood. Day after last treatment – "the best day I've had for years" and bowel movement regular again after many years.
20th (232 days)	Patient maintaining improved state of health.
21st (260 days)	Patient now enjoying good health – particularly sleeping well at night and has done so for past 2 weeks; through until 5/6am and **without having to urinate**.
22nd and last (298 days)	Patient declared that he had given himself one year to see what could be achieved. Left leg raised 15in. (38cm).

Patient remains happy and expressed gratitude.

Summary Outcome

- Alleviated frequent diarrhoea.
- Restored left leg gait – able to swing it and not drag it.
- Wear of toecap of left shoe ended.
- Ability to lift left leg 15in. (38.1cm) above horizontal, whilst sat, nil lift at outset.
- Sleeping soundly and undisturbed by need to urinate.
- Good health enjoyed and patient very grateful for progress made.
- Outcome not distorted by physiotherapy or occupational therapy – which had been withdrawn approximately 4 years before patient was seen.

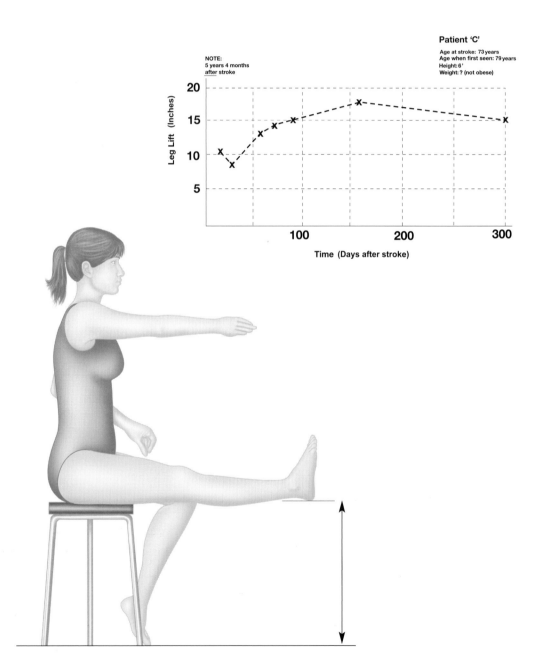

Patient 'C'

Age at stroke: 73 years
Age when first seen: 79 years
Height: 6'
Weight: ? (not obese)

NOTE:
5 years 4 months
after stroke

Leg Lift (Inches)

Time (Days after stroke)

Measurement used to assess and record progress of physical movement.

Stroke Patient Case Studies (Patient 'D')

Personal Details   Male, height 6'3" (1.90m), weight 17 stone (108kg).

Occupation   Retired veterinary practitioner.

Medical History   Age, at time of stroke, 77 years, 9 months.

Previously of good, robust, health. Phlegmatic personality.

Prostectomy 6 years before stroke. Stroke causing left side paralysis. Last 2 years – osteopathic treatment for back pain.

Medication

Paracetamol.

First Seen

Within first week of stroke and hospitalisation.

Presenting Signs / Symptoms / Information

• Left side hemiplegia.
• Patient bedridden initially.
• Tired, content to rest quietly.
• Patient complained of lower back pain.

Tender Areas of Feet at Initial Consultation

• Thyroid.
• Frontal and maxillary sinuses.
• Adrenals.
• Tail of pancreas.
• Right kidney.
• Left hip.
• T5/6 and L3/4 of spine.
• Coccyx area (left side biased).

Presenting Indications re. the Above

Lethargy (thyroid and adrenals – wife confirmed!). Congested sinuses suggested, 'thick' heads occasionally (patient confirmed). Possible discomfort, just above waist on right side. Back pain.

Patient's Aim

To regain as much mobility as possible.

Therapist's Aim

To reassure whilst 'telling it as it is', i.e. long course of treatment; patience and determination vital, etc. To regain as much mobility as possible and good body function.

Significant Events in Treatment Outcome

Hospital 42 days	) At 4th treatment (14 days)))) At 8th treatment) (35 days)	Spasm in paralysed left leg. Patient could feel sensation for first time. Patient feeling well: healthier complexion. Patient asleep by end of treatment – despite robust singing of Christmas carols on ward!
11th (49 days)		Left leg moved – slight upward move of knee (patient prone).
13th (56 days)		Patient raised left leg 1/2in. (13mm) above horizontal, at heel (patient prone).
15th (63 days)		Patient's previous constipation 'gone', after previous treatment. Left leg raised 11/2in. (37mm).
18th (75 days)		Left knee raised 21/2in. (75mm) above horizontal – patient prone. Got patient to 'pattern' movement, e.g. "1, 2 and raise" x 3 times – to build muscle co-ordination and strength.
19th (79 days)		Left knee raised 9in. (23cm) by patterned movement and 21/2in. (75mm) from static.
22nd (90 days)		Left knee raised 11in. (28cm) vertically; 31/2in. (9cm) from static.
30th (119 days)		Left leg lift 9in. (23cm) vertically, at heel, off bed (patient prone), can bend leg fully at knee and move leg medially, i.e. adduction of leg. Oedema of left foot and ankle.
35th (145 days)		Patient stood, supported on each side and holding head of bed. Stood for 30 seconds. Undone by fit of giggling.
37th (152 days)		Patient said left leg felt 'lighter', no longer a dead weight.
285 days		Patient stood (supported on each side) for 15 minutes uninterrupted. Viral infection; believed to have been brought by a well-meaning visitor.
59th (305 days)		Doctor checked blood pressure (normal).
60th (312 days)		Whilst worked extremely tender sigmoid flexure area, caused left leg to shoot back towards trunk! Working temporal / frontal of right side of brain. Left leg spasm. Repeated a number of times – to eliminate random chance reaction.

66th (354 days)	Patient stood for 5 minutes.
68th (368 days) & summary	Patient to move home in 6 days (re: house sale/relocation). Left leg very mobile. Patient stood for 5 minutes. Patient wheelchair bound during waking hours – seems philosophical, happy and content with his lot (wife's exhaustion a concern).

Note: There is no graphical representation of this patient's movement during treatment because the measurements contained in these notes were made with him prone on a bed. The other graphs refer to the patient seated (see page 152). Therefore, in that regard only, to include a graph for 'Patient D' would be a misleading distortion of the audit.

Strokes – Summary

The Audit covers four patients only but is intended to show the extent and limitations of reflexology used to complement the established procedures of occupational therapy and physiotherapy. In one case only (Patient C) the lapse of time of 6 years after the stroke meant that physiotherapy and occupational therapy had ceased 4 years previously. Any improvement would appear to be due to reflexology therapy.

The other aim of the audit (apart from the clarification and presentation of information held previously in the patients' records) is to encourage a much more exhaustive and thorough research into the potential benefit of including reflexology in a post-stroke treatment programme.

Whilst the small number within the audit limits any claim that would be significant, nevertheless it is hoped that it contributes a little to the understanding and treatment of this condition that can have such a dramatic and demoralising effect upon its sufferers.

Statistics: In all, 7 patients treated; 1 patient experienced a partial and small increase in the mobility of the affected arm; 2 patients showed no improvement after 7 treatments; 4 patients showed signs of increased mobility and restoration of an improved quality of life (as detailed per patient, i.e. 57%).

Factual Summary of General Situation in the UK

- A fifth of all stroke victims are under 40.
- By the time you have read this appendix, 5 more people will have had a stroke.
- One in three will have died.
- Strokes are the leading cause of severe disability.
- Strokes are the third most common cause of death in the Western world.
- Majority of those who survive a stroke will have a paralysed arm.
- Every year, 10,000 people of working age will suffer a stroke.
- Approximately a third, aged between 35 and 65, are unable to work again.
- The estimated cost in the UK is £2.8 billion each year.
- Up to 50% of patients suffer clinical depression.

A Positive View of the General Situation in the UK

These facts make depressing reading, so we will conclude this chapter by taking a positive view of the same data.

- 80% of the population under 40 are unlikely to have a stroke.
- By the time you have read this chapter only 5 people out of a population of some 58/60 million in the UK will have suffered a stroke.
- Of those, only one in three would have died and of those some would have been elderly.
- Strokes, whilst a major cause of severe disability, can be treated and, if caught early enough a full recovery is not unknown.
- Whilst strokes are the third most common cause of death in the Western world, severe adverse reaction to prescribed medication now ranks fourth and we are more likely to suffer a heart attack or a form of cancer.
- The majority of those who survive a stroke will have a paralysed arm but, otherwise, it is possible they will enjoy many more years of life of good quality.
- Approximately two thirds, between 35 and 65 are able to work again – even though some may die of boredom.
- The estimated cost in the UK of £2.8 billion is an incentive to take preventative measures to treat promptly and comprehensively.
- 50% of patients will not suffer clinical depression.

Too often we fall victim of news presentation that accentuates doom and gloom. Misfortune may be news in the media world, but those recovering from debilitating conditions need a positive, cheerful approach to life to aid their recovery.

Future Research

The considerable amount of unpaid time it took to produce the albeit limited Audit gives a reason why so little 'research' or validation studies of complementary therapies exists. Busy practitioners have insufficient time, in comparison to the research departments of University Medical Schools. This divergence needs addressing if sufficient and significant 'evidence-based' outcomes of complementary therapies is to be achieved.

Sources

The Stroke Association, London, EC1Y 8JJ.
'Different Strokes', London, E8 4QJ.
Personal 'hands-on' experience gained in working on patients in Bristol General Hospital, Weston-Super-Mare General Hospital (both UK) and in follow-up treatments.

Appendix to Book

Conditions That Responded to Reflexology Treatments

For the record, this summary was compiled from over 15 years of practice. It is not in any order of priority and, therefore, is in alphabetical order, simply for easy reference. They represent the conditions presented most frequently.

Allergies	Responded to general treatment, particularly to the endocrine system.
Back Pain	Most frequently lumbar and / or mid thoracic areas.
Blocked Ears	School-aged patients.
Bronchial Congestion	Often suspected adverse working environment.
Cancer	Bowel; cervical; always made it clear to patient and immediate relatives that the purpose was to make the quality of life as good as possible whilst they remained with us; no more and no less. Very humbling gratitude for what therapy was able to do for the patient.
Constipation	Often related to stress and frequently related to drinking insufficient water.
Debilitation	Put simply, no specific problem admitted other than 'the battery was run down'. Four treatments the norm, with significant improvement after three treatments – almost a "three treatment law".
Growth Problems	Children not as big, tall, as parent expected: child often apparently healthy and certainly active. Suspected parent anxiety rather than problem for the child. Encouraging results, however, from stimulating areas corresponding to the endocrine system – particularly pituitary.
Hay Fever	All patients responded positively; their gratitude lead to annual check-ups in April / May of each year – before high pollen counts. Adrenal area always tender.

Haemorrhoids	Reduction in discomfort (ache) achieved with all cases, after three treatments.
Irritable Bowel Syndrome (IBS)	Often anxiety based, excellent results in almost all cases.
Maintenance	Treatments given to 'the converted' – patients who, in the past, had experienced the benefits of reflexology and who wished to use the therapy to stay healthy and vigorous. Attended once every three, six or twelve months, according to individual need.
Migraine	Patients usually responded quickly and favourably. Again, increasing their intake of water proved to be a great help.
Multiple Sclerosis (MS)	Limited success, improvement (increased mobility) often plateaued. Outcome seemed to depend upon the attitude of the patient towards their illness.
Multiple Symptoms	This refers to a number of indications of constitutional imbalance and, therefore, requiring a general treatment to rebalance. In the majority of cases very successful; time and number of treatments to achieve sustained improvement in health proved variable. 'Rule of four treatments' often applied.
Nausea	Often vertigo but could also be an apparent neck problem. In one case it followed a previous whiplash injury that responded to treatment (four treatments).
Oedema (Lower Limbs)	Majority of patients had measured (using tape measure) reduced swelling. Can take five to six treatments to achieve definite benefit.
Pregnancy	Apparently helped patients conceive. Great success with pregnant, overdue, patients (within 48 hours) onset of labour and a natural birth; receipt of photograph of happy mum and smiling baby (probably wind!) often followed.
Sinus Congestion	Excellent, beneficial outcome for vast majority of patients.
Stress	No surprises here except a few directors of companies who attended as and when overcome by their responsibilities. This type of positive, in charge, person is often reluctant to admit the benefit to be gained from regular treatments of reflexology or similar therapies (usually a burst of three treatments was sufficient for all patients).
Strokes	see Chapter 7 and Appendix to Chapter 7.

Glossary of Terms and Medical Abbreviations

Contains terms not included in the index (*see* page 167).

ABDUCTION
movement of a bone away from the midline of the body (limb).

ADDUCTION
movement of a bone towards from the midline of the body (limb).

AMINO ACID
an organic chemical compound composed of one or more basic amino groups and one or more acidic carboxyl groups.

ANABOLISM
builds food molecules into larger, more complex molecule compounds and in so doing uses energy.

ANAEMIA
a decrease of haemoglobin in the blood to levels below the normal range of 4.2 million/mm^3 to 6.1 million/mm^3.

ANAESTHETICS
drugs or agents capable of producing a complete or partial loss of feeling (anaesthesia).

ANALGESIC
(i) relieving pain; (ii) a drug that relieves pain.

ANDROGENIC HORMONES
pertaining to the development of masculine characteristics.

ANTHRAX
a disease affecting primarily farm animals (cattle, goats, pigs, sheep and horses) caused by the bacterium *bacillus anthracis*. Humans get it from direct contact with infected animals or by inhalation of spores of the bacterium leading to a pulmonary form of the disease. Both forms are treatable with appropriate antibiotics.

ARRHYTHMIA
any deviation of the normal pattern of the heart beat.

ASTHMA
a respiratory disorder characterised by recurring episodes or attacks of difficulty in breathing / restricted breathing and wheezing on expiration / inspiration caused by constriction of the bronchi, coughing and viscous mucoid bronchial secretions.

ASTRINGENT
a substance that causes contraction of tissues upon application.

ATAXIA
an abnormal condition characterised by impaired ability to co-ordinate movement, e.g. a staggering gait or postural imbalance.

ATOPIC
pertaining to a hereditary tendency to experience immediate allergic reactions (such as asthma, atopic dermatitis) because of the presence of an antibody in the skin and sometimes in the bloodstream.

ATRIUM
a chamber or cavity, as in the left and right atria of the heart, or the nasal cavity.

AUTOIMMUNE
pertaining to the development of an immune response to one's own tissues.

BERIBERI
a disease of peripheral nerves caused by a deficiency or an inability to assimilate thiamine.

BIOELECTRONIC
pertaining to electrical current that is generated by living tissues, such as nerves and muscles.

BOWEN TECHNIQUE
a series of gentle, rolling, moves on the muscle and connective tissue along the whole body, using the thumb and fingers on precise areas with no more pressure than could be applied to the eyeball, for example, without discomfort.

CARBOHYDRATE
a group of organic compounds, the most important of which are the saccharides, starch, glucose and glycogen.

CARBUNCLE
a large site of staphylococcal infection containing purulent matter in deep, interconnecting subcutaneous pockets.

CARDIAC PLEXUS
one of several nerve clusters situated close to the arch of the aorta.

CALCANEUS
heel bone of the foot.

CAROTID
pertaining to the arteries that supply blood to the head and neck.

CATABOLISM
a metabolic process in which complex substances are broken down by living cells into simple compounds. The process produces carbon dioxide and water and releases energy for work, energy-storage or heat production[2].

CATALYST
a substance that influences the rate of chemical reaction without being altered permanently or being consumed by the process.

CATARACT
an abnormal progressive condition of the lens of the eye characterised by loss of transparency. A grey-white opacity that can be observed within the lens behind the pupil.

CEREBELLUM
part of the brain located in the posterior cranial fossa behind the brainstem.

CEREBRAL CORTEX
a layer or neurons and synapses (grey matter) on the surface of the cerebral hemispheres and folds. About two thirds of its area is buried in fissures.

CERVICAL GANGLIA
a cluster of neurons associated with a network of nerves formed by the ventral primary divisions of the first four cervical nerves of the eight pairs of nerves of the neck between the atlas and the seventh vertebrae.

CHLOROFORM
a non-flammable volatile liquid; the first inhalation anaesthetic to be discovered. It has a low margin of safety and significant toxicity. The drug is not used in the United States.

CHOLERA
an acute bacterial infection of the small intestine characterised by severe diarrhoea and vomiting, muscular cramps, dehydration and depletion of electrolytes.

COELIAC DISEASE
a condition characterised by an intolerance of gluten.

COLITIS
an inflammatory condition of the large intestine characterised by severe diarrhoea, bleeding and ulceration of the mucosa of the intestine.

COLLAGEN
a protein consisting of bundles of tiny reticular fibrils that combine to form the white glistening, inelastic, fibres of the tendons, ligaments and fascia.

CONJUNCTIVITIS
inflammation of the conjunctiva (mucous membrane lining the inner surfaces of the eyelid and interior part of the sclera). It is caused by bacterial or viral infection, allergy or environmental factors.

CRAMP
a spasmodic and often painful contraction of one or more muscles.

CUBOID BONE
a tarsal bone on the lateral side of the foot, proximal to the fourth and fifth metatarsal bones.

CUNEIFORM BONES
three wedge-shaped tarsal bones of the foot medial to the cuboid bone.

DIABETES MELLITUS (DM)
a complex disorder of carbohydrates, fat and protein metabolism that is primarily a result of a deficiency or complete lack of insulin secretion by the beta cells of the pancreas, or of defects of the insulin receptors.

DIPHTHERIA
an acute, contagious, disease caused by the bacterium *corynebacterium diphtheriae*.

DORSIFLEXION
in relation to the foot, bending the upper surface of the foot back towards the body.

EFFICACY
the maximum ability of a drug or treatment to produce a result, regardless of dosage.

ELECTROCARDIOGRAPH (ECG)
a device used for recording the electrical activity of the myocardium to detect transmission of the cardiac impulse through the conductive tissue of the muscle of the heart.

ELECTROENCEPHALOGRAM (EEG)
a graphic chart on which is traced the electrical potential produced by the brain cells, as detected by electrodes placed on the scalp.

ELECTROMYOGRAPHY (EMG)
a record of the intrinsic electrical activity in a skeletal muscle at rest.

EMBOLISM
an abnormal circulatory condition in which a foreign body travels through the bloodstream and becomes lodged in a blood vessel.

EMBOLUS
a foreign object, quantity of air or gas, a piece of tissue or tumour or a piece of thrombus that circulates in the bloodstream until it becomes lodged in a vessel.

EPILEPSY
a group of neurological disorders characterised by recurrent episodes of convulsive seizures, sensory disturbances, abnormal behaviour, loss of consciousness, or all of these.

EVERSION
turning the sole of the foot outward.

FARADIC PAD
a pad through which a low electrical current can be passed for a specific time and on a particular part of the body, as used in physiotherapy and chiropody (podiatry).

FASCIA
fibrous connective tissue of the body that may be separated from other specifically organised structures, such as tendons and ligaments. It varies in thickness and density and in the amount of fat, collagenous fibre, elastic fibre and tissue fluid it contains.

FIBROCYSTIC
the presence of single or multiple cysts that are palpable in the breasts.

FIBULA
the lateral bone of the lower leg.

FLATUS
air or gas in the intestine that is passed out through the rectum.

FOLLICLE
(i) a pouch depression, such as the dental follicles that enclose the teeth before eruption or the hair follicles within the epidermis; (ii) fluid or colloid-filled ball of cells in some glands such as the thyroid.

GANGRENE
necrosis or death of tissue, usually from the loss of blood supply, bacterial invasion and subsequent putrefaction. The extremities are affected usually but it can occur in the intestines and gallbladder.

GLAUCOMA
an abnormal condition of elevated pressure within the eye.

GLYCOSIDE
any of several carbohydrates that yield a sugar and a non-sugar on hydrolysis. The plant *digitalis purpurea* yields a glycoside used in the treatment of heart disease.

GOITRE
an enlarged thyroid gland, usually evident as a pronounced swelling in the neck.

GOUT
a disease associated with an inborn error of uric acid metabolism that increases production or interferes with the secretion of uric acid. Excess uric acid is converted to sodium urate crystals that precipitate from the blood and become deposited in joints and other tissues.

HALLUX
large or great toe.

HEPATITIS
an inflammatory condition of the liver, characterised by jaundice, clay-coloured stools and tea-coloured urine. May be caused by bacterial or viral infection, parasitic infection, alcohol, drugs, toxins or transfusion of incompatible blood.

HIATUS HERNIA
protrusion of a portion of the stomach upwards through the diaphragm. The condition is said to occur in approximately 40% of the population.

HISTAMINE
a compound found in all cells, produced by the breakdown of histidine (an amino acid found in many proteins). It is released in allergic inflammatory conditions and causes dilation of capillaries, decrease in blood pressure, increase in secretion of gastric juice and constriction of smooth muscles of the bronchi and uterus.

HOMOEOPATHY
a system of therapeutics based on the theory that 'like cures like' as advanced in the late 18th century by Dr. Samuel Hahnemann.

HYDROCELE
an accumulation of fluid in any sack-like cavity or duct – specifically in the tunica vaginalis, testis or along the spermatic cord.

HYPERTHYROIDISM
hyperactivity of the thyroid gland which is enlarged usually. It secretes greater than normal amounts of thyroid hormones and the metabolic process of the body is accelerated.

HYPOGLYCAEMIA
less than the normal amount of glucose in the blood, usually caused by the administration of too much insulin, excessive secretion of insulin by the islet cells of the pancreas, or dietary deficiency.

HYPOKALAEMIA
a condition in which there is an abnormally low quantity of potassium circulating in the bloodstream.

IMPETIGO
a streptococcal, staphylococcal or combined infection of the skin. Characterised by discrete fragile vesicles with an erythematous border. Becomes pustular. Lesions form usually on the face and spread locally. The disorder is highly contagious through contact with the discharge from the lesions.

INFARCTION
the development of an infarct which includes myocardial infarction ('heart attack') and pulmonary infarction.

INFARCT
a localised area of necrosis in a tissue, vessel, organ or part.

INOCULATION
the process of introducing a substance (inoculum) into the body to produce or to increase immunity to the disease or condition associated with the substance.

INSULIN
(i) a naturally occurring hormone secreted by the beta cells of the Islets of Langerhans in the pancreas in response to increased levels of glucose in the blood; (ii) a pharmacological preparation of the hormone administered in treating diabetes mellitus.

KERATIN
a fibrous sulphur containing protein that is the primary component of the epidermis, hair, nails, enamel of the teeth and horny tissue of animals.

KERATOLYSIS
the loosening and shedding of the outer layer of the skin.

LATERAL
away from the midline of the body.

LIPASE
any of several enzymes produced by the organs of the digestive system that catalyze the breakdown of lipids through the hydrolysis of the linkages between fatty acids and glycerol in triglycerides and phospholipids.

LUMBAR
pertaining to the part of the body between the thorax and the pelvis.

MACROPHAGE
any cell capable of engulfing other cells and debris in the tissues. Part of a widely scattered system of cells fulfilling vital functions, particularly in the liver and spleen.

MALLEOLUS
a rounded bony process such as the protuberance on each side of the ankle.

MASTITIS
in inflammatory condition of the breast, usually caused by streptococcal or staphylococcal infection.

MELANIN
a black or dark brown pigment that occurs naturally in the skin, hair and iris of the eye.

METABOLISM
the aggregate of all chemical processes that occur in living organisms, resulting in growth, generation of energy, elimination of wastes and other body functions as they relate to the distribution of nutrients in the blood after digestion.

MITOCHONDRIA
a small rod-like, thread-like granular organelle within the cytoplasm that functions in cellular metabolism and respiration and occurs in varying numbers in all living cells except bacteria, viruses, blue-green algae and mature erythrocytes.

MITRAL VALVE
a bicuspid valve situated between the left atrium and the left ventricle; the only valve with two rather than three cusps.

MUCILAGE
a sticky mixture of carbohydrates produced by plant cell activity.

MYXOEDEMA
the most severe form of hypothyroidism (low thyroid function). It is characterised by swelling of the hands, feet, face and area surrounding the eye sockets (periorbital tissue).

NEURALGIA
an abnormal condition characterised by severe stabbing pain, caused by a variety of disorders affecting the nervous system.

OBSTETRICS
a branch of medicine concerned with pregnancy and childbirth.

OCCIPITAL
pertaining to the occipital bone – a cup-like bone at the back of the head.

OEDEMA
the abnormal accumulation of fluid in interstitial spaces of tissues.

OSTEOMALACIA
an abnormal condition of the bone characterised by loss of calcification of the matrix resulting in softening of the bone, weakness, fracture, pain, anorexia and weight-loss.

OSTEOPATHS
practitioners who recognise and correct structural problems using massage and manipulation. The process is important in both the diagnosis and treatment of health problems.

OSTEOPOROSIS
a disorder characterised by abnormal loss of bone density.

PARATHYROID GLAND
any of several small structures, usually four, attached to the dorsal surfaces of the lateral lobes of the thyroid gland.

PELLAGRA
a disease resulting from a deficiency of niacin or tryptophan or a metallic defect that interferes with the conversion of the precursor tryptophan to niacin. Commonly seen in people whose diet primarily consists of maize. Shows as scaly dermatitis.

PEPSIN
an enzyme secreted in the stomach that catalyzes the hydrolysis of protein.

PEPTIC
pertaining to the digestion or to the enzymes or secretions essential to digestion.

PHYSIOTHERAPIST
a person licensed in the examination, testing and treatment of physical impairments through the use of special exercise, application of heat or cold and other physical modalities.

PINEAL GLAND
a cone-shaped structure in the brain. Its precise function has not been established. It may secrete a hormone melatonin which appears to inhibit the secretion of luteinizing hormone.

PITUITARY GLAND
a endocrine gland suspended beneath the brain, in the sella turcica and covered by an extension of the duramater, called the pituitary diaphragm. It is divided into an anterior adenohypophysis and a smaller posterior neurohypophysis. It is the 'conductor' of the endocrine system, secreting many hormones via a balancing feed-back system.

PLACEBO EFFECT
a physical or emotional change occurring after a substance is taken or administered that is not the result of any property of the substance.

PLANTAR FLEXION
bending of the under side of the foot down away from the body.

POLYSACCHARIDE
a carbohydrate that contains three or more molecules of simple carbohydrates, e.g. starches, glycogens and cellulose.

PROSTATE
a gland in men that surrounds the neck of the bladder and the deepest part of the urethra and produces a secretion that liquefies coagulated semen.

PROSTATITIS
acute or chronic inflammation of the prostate gland, with or without swelling.

PRURITIC
pertaining to itching accompanied by the urge to scratch.

PULMONARY VEIN
one of two pairs of large vessels that return oxygenated blood from each lung to the left atrium of the heart.

PYORRHOEA
(i) discharge of pus; (ii) a purulent inflammation of the tissues surrounding the teeth.

RABIES
an acute (usually fatal) viral disease of the central nervous system of animals. Transmitted from animals to people by infected blood, tissue or, mostly, by saliva.

RAYNAUD'S DISEASE
intermittent attacks of ischaemia of the extremities of the body, especially the fingers, toes, ears and nose, caused by exposure to cold or by emotional stimuli.

REFLEXOLOGY
is a technique based upon the principle that there are areas on the feet and hands that correspond to all the glands, organs and parts of the body. It is a unique method of using the thumb and fingers on these areas to encourage the body's innate ability to heal itself and to produce homoeostatis.

RENIN
a proteolytic enzyme (any substance that promotes the breakdown of protein).

RHEUMATISM
(i) any of a large number of inflammatory conditions of the bursae, joints, ligaments or muscles characterised by pain, limitation of movement and structural degeneration of simple or multiple parts of the musculo-skeletal system; (ii) the syndrome of pain, limitation of movement and structural degeneration of elements in the musculo-skeletal system as may occur in gout, rheumatoid arthritis, and many other diseases.

RICKETS
a condition caused by the deficiency of Vitamin D primarily in infancy and characterised by abnormal bone formation.

SACRAL
pertaining to the sacrum – the large triangular bone at the dorsal part of the pelvis inserted like a wedge between the two hipbones.

SAPONIN
a soapy material found in some plants, especially soapwart and certain lilies. Generally, have been replaced by synthetic preparations.

SARCOIDOSIS
a chronic disorder of unknown origin characterised by the formation of tubercles (nodules).

SCLEROSIS
a condition characterised by hardening of tissue resulting from any of several causes, including inflammation, the deposit of mineral salts and inflammation of connective tissue fibres.

SCIATICA
inflammation of the sciatic nerve usually marked by pain and tenderness along the course of the nerve, from the lower back, through the thigh and down the leg.

SEBORRHOEIC
referring to any of several skin conditions in which an overproduction of sebum results in excessive oiliness or dry scales.

SMALLPOX
a highly contagious viral disease characterised by fever, and a vesicular, pustular rash.

STEVENS–JOHNSON SYNDROME
a serious, sometimes fatal, inflammatory disease affecting children and young adults.

STREPTOCOCCAL
pertaining to any of the species of the bacterium *streptococcus*.

SUBARACHNOID
space around the brain and spinal cord; filled with cerebrospinal fluid which acts as a protective cushion to the brain and spinal cord.

SUBCUTANEOUS
beneath the skin.

SYNTHESIS
combining form meaning 'putting together or formation of', e.g. the synthesis of Vitamin D from sunlight.

TACHYCARDIA
a condition in which the myocardium contracts at a rate greater than 100 beats per minute.

TALUS BONE
the second largest tarsal bone. It supports the tibia and rests on the calcaneus.

TANNIN
a substance obtained from the bark and fruit of various trees and shrubs.

TARTRATES
from tartaric acid; a colourless or white powder found in various plants.

TRIPLE HEATER (SANJIAO)
a yang concept consisting of openings to the stomach, small intestine and bladder, together forming an energy system concerned with the free flow of fluids and nutrients.

TUBERCULOSIS (TB)
a chronic granulomatous infection caused by acid-fast bacillus, *mycobacterium tuberculosis*. Generally, it is transmitted by inhalation or ingestion of infected droplets that affects the lungs, although infection of multiple organ systems occurs.

UREA
a systemic osmotic diuretic and topical keratolytic.

VENTRICLE
a small cavity, such as the right and left ventricle of the heart or one of the cavities filled with cerebrospinal fluid in the brain.

WEIL'S DISEASE
most serious form of the disease leptospirosis which is very infectious and is transmitted by the urine of wild or domestic animals – especially rats and dogs. Weil's Disease is known also as '*Autumn Fever*'.

WOLFF-PARKINSON-WHITE SYNDROME
a disorder of the atrioventricular (AV) conduction, characterised by two AV conduction pathways.

XEROPHTHALMIA
condition of dry and lusterless corneas and conjunctival areas of the eye, usually the result of a Vitamin A deficiency and associated with night blindness.

The following is not a comprehensive list of medical abbreviations. Abbreviations in common use can vary from place to place. Each countries' or institution's list should be used as the authority for their acceptable abbreviations.

Ab	antibody
ACTH	adrenocorticotropic hormone
ADH	antidiuretic hormone
ADL	activities of daily living
ADR	adverse drug reaction
AF	atrial fibrillation
AIDS	acquired immunodeficiency syndrome
aj	ankle jerk
AK	above-knee
a.m.a	against medical advice
ARD	acute respiratory disease
Bact.	**L.** bacterium
Bib	drink
b.i.d.	twice a day (**L.** bis in die)
BK	below-knee
Bl	blood
BMR	basal metabolic rate
BMI	body mass index
BP	blood pressure
bpm	beats per minute (re: pulse)
CABS	coronary artery bypass surgery
CBC	complete blood count
CHD	coronary (congenital) heart disease
CNS	central nervous system
c/o	complains of
CPR	cardiopulmonary resuscitation
CS	caesarean section
CSF	cerebrospinal fluid
CVA	cerebrovascular accident ("stroke")
CXR	chest X-ray
d	day; **L.** diem
D&C	dilation and curettage

DM	diabetes mellitus
DOB	date of birth
DNA	did not attend (*also* deoxyribonucleic acid but much less common use)
DVT	deep venous thrombosis
ECG	electrocardiogram
EEG	electroencephalogram
EMS	emergency medical service
ENT	ear, nose, and throat
ESR	erythrocyte sedimentation rate
FB	foreign body
FH	family history
FSH	follicule-stimulating hormone
ft	foot
GH	growth hormone
GI	gastrointestinal
GP	general practitioner
H&P	history and physical
Hb or Hgb	haemoglobin
HEENT	head, eye, ear, nose, and throat
HIV	human immunodeficiency virus
h/o	history of
HR	heart rate ("pulse")
HT; HTN	hypertension ("high BP")
I	iodine (re: thyroid function)
ICU	intensive care unit
IDDM	insulin-dependent diabetes mellitus
IV	intravenous
Kj	knee jerk
KUB	kidney, ureter, and bladder
L	left; lumbar; lung; length; lethal
LH	luteinizing hormone
lig.	ligament
LMP	last menstrual period
LNMP	last normal menstrual period
LP	lumbar puncture
mcg; μg	microgram
mg	milligram
MI	myocardial infarction ("heart attack")
MRI	magnetic resonance imaging
MS	multiple sclerosis
MVA	motor vehicle accident (in UK; RTA – road traffic accident)
n	normal
NAD	no appreciable disease
n.b.	not well
NIDDM	non-insulin-dependent diabetes mellitus
NKA	no known allergies
NSAID	nonsteroidal antiinflammatory drug
OB	obstetrics
OT	occupational therapy

PH	past history
PMS	premenstrual syndrome
PO; p.o.	orally; by mouth (**L.** per os)
ppm	parts per million
PSA	prostate-specific antigen
q.	every, each (**L.** quaque)
q.d.	every day (**L.** quaque die)
RA	rheumatoid arthritis
RAI	radioactive iodine
RBC; rbc	red blood cell; red blood count
RDA	recommended daily / dietary allowance
ROM	range of motion; range of movement
S.	sacral vertebrae
SLE	systemic lupus erythematosus
SOB	shortness of breath
s/s	signs and symptoms
STD	sexually transmitted disease
Sx	symptoms
T_3	triiodothyronine (re: thyroid function)
T_4	thyroxine
t.d.s.	to be taken three times a day (**L.** ter die sumendum)
TB	tuberculosis; tubercle bacillus; tuberculin
TENS	transcutaneous electrical nerve stimulation
TIA	transient ischaemic attack
TMJ	temporomandibular joint
TPR	temperature, pulse, and respiration
TSH	thyroid-stimulating hormone
TST	triple sugar iron test
Tx	treatment
UA	urinalysis
URI	upper respiratory infection
US	ultrasound
UTI	urinary tract infection
VD	venereal disease
Vf	visual field
WBC; wbc	white blood cell; white blood count
wt	weight
yo	years old

References

1. Glanze, W. D. (ed.): 1998. *Mosby's Medical, Nursing, and Allied Health Dictionary*, 5th Edition. Mosby, London. (ISBN: 0 8151 4800 3).
2. Warrier, G., and Gunawant, D.: 1997. *The Complete Illustrated Guide to Ayurveda: The Ancient Indian Healing Tradition*. Element, UK. (ISBN: 1 85230 952 0).
3. Anthony, C. P. 1983: *Textbook of Anatomy and Physiology*. Mosby, London. (ISBN: 0 8016 0289 0).
4. Webster's. 1980. *New Webster's Dictionary – Encyclopedic Edition*. Delair Publ., USA. (ISBN: 0 8326 0001 6).

Useful Addresses

Reflexology

Ann Gillanders
Healing Points
BS Reflexology Sales
92 Sheering Road
Old Harlow, Essex, CM17 0JW, UK
Tel: 44 (0) 1279 429060
E-mail: info@footreflexology.com
Web: www.footreflexology.com

International Council of Reflexologists
P O Box 78060
Westcliffe Postal Outlet
Hamilton, ON L9C 7N5
Ontario, Canada
Tel: 00 (1) 905 387 8449
E-mail: icr@mountaincable.net
Web: www.icr-reflexology.org

International Institute of Reflexology®
Head Office
P O Box 12642
St. Petersburg
Florida 33733–2642, USA
Tel: 00 (1) 727 343 4811
E-mail: iir@tampabay.rr.com
Web: www.reflexology-usa.net

UK Head Office
146 Upperthorpe
Walkley, Sheffield
South Yorkshire, S6 3NF, UK
Tel: 44 (0) 1142 812100
E-mail: info@reflexology-uk.net
Web: www.reflexology-uk.net

Reflexology in Europe Network (RIEN)
Bovenover 59
1025 JJ Amsterdam
The Netherlands
Tel: 00 (31) 20 636 3915
E-mail: h.van.der.werff@freeler.nl
Web: www.reflexeurope.org

Reflexology Forum
P.O. Box 2367
South Croydon, Surrey, CR2 7ZE, UK
Tel: 44 (0800) 0370130

Association of Reflexologists
27 Old Gloucester Street,
London, WC1N 3XX, UK
Tel: 44 (0) 870 567 3320
E-mail: info@aor.org.uk
Web: www.aor.org.uk

ART (Advanced Reflexology Training)
Director: Mr. Anthony Porter
28 Hollyfield Avenue, London, N11 3BY, UK
Tel: 44 (0) 208 368 0865
E-mail: artreflex@btinternet.com
Web: www.artreflex.com

Booth VRT (Vertical Reflex Therapy) Ltd.
Suite 205
60 Westbury Hill, Bristol, BS9 3UJ, UK
Tel: 44 (0) 117 9626746
E-mail: contact@boothvrt.com
Web: www.boothvrt.com

Manual Neuro-Therapy & Neuro-Reflexology
Director: Nico Pauly
IRSK-WINGS
Oude Veurnestratt 75
8900 Leper
Belgium
Tel: (00) 32 57 33 60 83
E-mail: irsk-wings@itinera.be

Nutrition

Many of the following companies provide
professional advice and seminars that enable
therapists to expand their knowledge or keep
up-to-date, in addition to supplying their
supplementary products.

Biocare Ltd.
Lakeside
180 Lifford Lane
Kings Norton, Birmingham, B30 3NU, UK
Tel: 44 (0) 121 433 3727
E-mail: biocare@biocare.co.uk
Web: www.biocare.co.uk

An independent, science-based company
founded by practitioners with many years'
experience in biological science and nutrition.

Bioforce (UK) Ltd.
2 Brewster Place
Irvine, Scotland, KA11 5DD
Tel: 44 (0) 294 277 344
E-mail: enquiries@bioforce.co.uk
Web: www.bioforce.co.uk

Enzyme Process (UK)
Broadgate House
Westlode Street, Spalding, Lincolnshire
PE11 2AF, UK
Tel: 44 (0) 845 1300 776

Health care practitioners only or by
prescription.

Lamberts Healthcare Ltd.
Century Place
Lamberts Road, Tunbridge Wells, Kent
TN2 3EH, UK
Tel: 44 (0) 1892 552121

Health care practitioners only or by
prescription.

Nutri Ltd.
Meridian House
Botany Business Park, Whaley Bridge
High Peak, SK23 7DQ, UK
Tel: 44 (0) 1663 718 850
E-mail: webmaster@nutri.co.uk
Web: www.nutri.co.uk

Potters Herbal Medicines
Leyland Mill Lane
Wigan, Lancashire, WN1 2SB, UK

Solgar Vitamins Ltd.
Beggar's Lane, Aldbury
Tring, Herts, HP23 5PT, UK
Tel: 44 (0) 1442 890 355
E-mail: solgarinfo@solgar.com
Web: www.solgar.com

The Dr. Edward Bach Centre
Mount Vernon, Brightwell-cum-Sotwell
Wallingford, Oxfordshire, OX10 0PZ, UK
Tel: 44 (0) 1491 834 678
Web: www.bachcentre.com

The Nutri Centre
7 Park Crescent
London, W1B 1PF, UK
Tel: 44 (0) 207 436 5122
E-mail: customerservices@nutricentre.com
Web: www.nutricentre.com

Energy

Energy Works
Directors: Anna Jeoffroy & Philip Salmon
P.O. Box 145
Potters Bar
Hertfordshire, EN6 1TY, UK
Tel: 44 (0) 1707 657 577
E-mail: enquiries@energyworks.co.uk
Web: www.energyworks.co.uk

Workshops on Body Energy book: *Dr. Bach's
Flower Remedies & the Chakras*

Electronic Medicine Association
UK Director: John Morley-Kirk, FEMA
The Other End
1 Dragon Street, Granby
Nottinghamshire, NG13 9PN, UK
Tel: 44 (0) 1949 850068
E-mail: jmk@electronicmed.freeserve.co.uk
Web: www.electronicmed.com

In the USA
409 Marquette Drive, Louisville
KY40 222, USA
Tel: 00 (1) 502 423 1188
E-mail: holistic@aol.com

The British Acupuncture Council
63 Jeddo Road
London, W12 9HQ, UK
Tel: 44 (0) 208 735 0400
E-mail: info@acupuncture.org.uk
Web: www.acupuncture.org.uk

Ayurvedic Company of Great Britain Ltd.
50 Penywern Road
London, SW5 9SX, UK

Lilian Tibshraeny-Morten
Director, JLM Educational Training
Reflexology & Meridian Therapy
15462 Gulf Blvd #906
Madeira Beach
FL 33708, USA
Tel: 091 (727) 319 6818
E-mail: lilian@reflexologyusa.com
Web: www.reflexologyusa.com

Book: *Moving The Energy – Reflexology and Meridian Therapy – Introducing the Wand Reflex Method.*

Jan de Vries
Healthcare Ltd.
Auchenkyle
Southwood Road, Troon
Ayrshire, KA10 7EL, Scotland
Tel: 44 (0) 1292 311414
E-mail: info@jandevrieshealth.co.uk
Web: www.jandevrieshealth.co.uk

Physiotherapy / Osteopathy

Chartered Society of Physiotherapy
14 Bedford Row
London, WC1R 4ED, UK
Tel: 44 (0) 207 306 6666
E-mail: enquiries@csp.org.uk
Web: www.csp.org.uk

General Osteopathic Council
Osteopathy House
176 Tower Bridge Road
London, SE1 3LU, UK
Tel: 44 (0) 207 357 6655
E-mail: info@osteopathy.org.uk
Web: www.osteopathy.org.uk

The Northern Institute of Massage
14–16 St. Mary's Place
Bury, Lancashire, BL9 0DZ, UK
Tel: 44 (0) 161 797 1800
E-mail: information@nim.co.uk
Web: www.nim.co.uk

Register of Remedial Masseurs & Manipulative Therapies
330 Lytham Road, Blackpool, FY4 1DW, UK
Tel: 44 (0) 1253 408443
E-mail: admin.lcsp@ic24.net
Web: www.lcsp.uk.com

Training leads to qualification by a progressive series of written and practical examinations to Membership of the LCSP.

Research

Medical Research Council (MRC)
20 Park Crescent
London, W1N 1AL, UK
Tel: 44 (0) 207 636 5422
E-mail:
firstname.surname@headoffice.mrc.ac.uk
Web: www.mrc.ac.uk

Research Council for Complementary Medicine
60 Great Ormond Street
London, WC1N 3JF, UK
Tel: 44 (0) 207 833 8897

Centre for Complementary Health Studies
University of Exeter
Amory Building
Exeter, EX4 4RJ, UK
Tel: 44 (0) 1392 661000
Web: www.ex.ac.uk

Lancaster University
Bailrigg
Lancaster, LA1 4YW, UK
Tel: 44 (0) 1524 65201
Web: www.lancs.ac.uk

University of Manchester
Oxford Road
Manchester, M13 9PL, UK
Tel: 44 (0) 161 306 6000
Web: www.manchester.ac.uk

University of Southampton
University Road
Highfield, Southampton, SO17 1BJ, UK
Tel: 44 (0) 23 8079 5000
Web: www.soton.ac.uk

University of Westminster
Headquarters
309 Regent Street
London, W1B 2UW, UK
Tel: 44 (0) 20 7911 5000
Web: www.wmin.ac.uk

Strokes

The Stroke Association
Stroke House
Whitecross Street
London, EC1Y 8JJ, UK

Response to Audit. Quote from Chief Executive: "*I have passed details of this on to colleagues working in this field of research.*"
Different Strokes
Sir Walter Scott House
2 Broadway Market
London, E8 4QJ, UK

Response to Audit. Quote from Director: "*Thanks for useful presentation. We will put it to the best use we can.*" Also enclosed with response, was a copy of their annual review and a copy of their latest newsletter.

Additional Useful Addresses

British Medical Association (BMA)
BMA House
Tavistock Square
London, WC1H 9JP, UK
Tel: 44 (0) 207 387 4499
E-mail: info.web@bma.org.uk
Web: www.bma.org.uk

General Medical Council (GMC)
Regent's Place
350 Euston Road
London, NW1 3JN, UK
Tel: 44 (0) 8453 578001
E-mail: gmc@gmc-uk.org
Web: www.gmc-uk.org

Royal College of General Practitioners
14 Princes Gate
Hyde Park
London, SW7 1PU, UK
Tel: 44 (0) 207 581 3232
E-mail: info@rcgp.org.uk
Web: www.rcgp.org.uk

Index